Springer Series on Geriatric Nursing

Mathy D. Mezey, RN, EdD, FAAN, Series Editor
New York University Division of Nursing

Advisory Board: Margaret Dimond, PhD, RN, FAAN; Steven H. Ferris, PhD; Terry Fulmer, RN, PhD, FAAN; Linda Kaeser, PhD, RN, ACSW, FAAN; Virgene Kayser-Jones, PhD, RN, FAAN; Eugenia Siegler, MD; Neville E. Strumpf, PhD, RN, FAAN; May Wykle, PhD, RN, FAAN; Mary K. Walker, PhD, RN, FAAN

WY 152 BAR £42.50

369 0299655

Bathing With a Battle

MONKLANDS HOSPITAL
LIBRARY

Person-Directed Care of Individuals With Dementia

Second Edition

WY 152 BAR £42.50

MONKLANDS HOSPITAL
LIBRARY
MONKSCOURT AVENUE
AIRDRIE ML60JS
☎01236712005

Ann Louise Barrick, PhD, is a clinical professor at the University of North Carolina-Chapel Hill, Department of Psychology, and director of psychology at John Umstead Hospital, Butner, North Carolina. She holds a doctorate in counseling psychology from Ball State University and has been a geropsychologist since 1986. She provides training to professional staff in the assessment and treatment of persons with dementia. She has conducted research and published articles addressing behavioral symptoms in dementia and is coauthor of two training films and a CD/DVD on methods for bathing persons with dementia.

Joanne Rader, RN, MN, is currently an independent consultant. She has worked in the field of long-term care for 30 years. She has worked on funded projects to reduce the use of physical restraints, inappropriate psychoactive medications, and defensive, self-protective behaviors during bathing and morning care for persons with dementia. She is the author of a 1996 AJN Book of the Year titled *Individualized Dementia Care: Creative, Compassionate Approaches.* She has published numerous articles and books addressing the emotional needs and behavioral symptoms of persons with dementia and has co-authored and produced manuals and videos on individualized wheelchair seating for older adults. She is a founding member and board member of the Pioneer Network, an organization working to change the culture of aging in the United States.

Beverly Hoeffer, DNSc, RN, FAAN, is professor and associate dean emerita, School of Nursing, Oregon Health and Science University in Portland, Oregon. She received her master's degree in advanced psychiatric nursing from Rutgers University and her doctorate in nursing science from the University of California, San Francisco. She is a member of the Western Academy of Nurses and a fellow in the American Academy of Nursing. Her research focused on behavioral symptoms of dementia, including outcome measures and clinical interventions for bathing persons with dementia, for over 20 years. Dr. Hoeffer has made numerous presentations and has authored articles and book chapters on the care of persons with dementia.

Philip D. Sloane, MD, MPH, is Elizabeth and Oscar Goodwin Distinguished Professor of Family Medicine at the University of North Carolina at Chapel Hill. A geriatrician, he has served as medical director for several long-term care facilities and has coauthored *Primary Care Geriatrics, Dementia Units in Long-Term Care,* and the Alzheimer's Association's *Key Elements of Dementia Care.* Dr. Sloane is nationally known for his work on the management of persons with Alzheimer's disease and related disorders.

Stacey Biddle, COTA/L, has combined her creative talents with degrees in art therapy and occupational therapy by providing direct services for 15 years to seniors in skilled, long-term assisted living, outpatient, home health care, and health care travel assignment. She has extensive experience adapting and modifying the environment to enhance the quality of life and daily living activities of older adults. In addition, Ms. Biddle has applied her expertise through publication and project management of research on HIV, dementia, adapted wardrobe systems, and incontinence studies.

Bathing Without a Battle

Person-Directed Care of Individuals With Dementia

Second Edition

Ann Louise Barrick, *PhD*

Joanne Rader, *RN, MN*

Beverly Hoeffer, *DNSc, RN, FAAN*

Philip D. Sloane, *MD, MPH*

Stacey Biddle, *COTA/L*

Editors

SPRINGER PUBLISHING COMPANY

New York

Copyright © 2008 Springer Publishing Company, LLC

All rights reserved.

No part of this publication may be reproduced, stored in a retrieval system, or
transmitted in any form or by any means, electronic, mechanical, photocopying,
recording, or otherwise, without the prior permission of Springer Publishing
Company, LLC.

Springer Publishing Company, LLC
11 West 42nd Street
New York, NY 10036–8002
www.springerpub.com

Acquisitions Editor: Allan Graubard
Production Editor: Shana Meyer
Cover Design: Mimi Flow
Composition: Aptara Inc.

07   08   09   10   /   5   4   3   2   1

Library of Congress Cataloging-in-Publication Data

Bathing without a battle : person-directed care of individuals with dementia / Ann Louise
Barrick ... [et al., editors]. – 2nd ed.
     p. ; cm. – (Springer series on geriatric nursing)
   Includes bibliographical references and index.
   ISBN 978-0-8261-0124-2 (pbk.)
  1. Dementia–Patients–Care.   2. Dementia–Patients–Services for.   3. Baths.   4. Older
people–Health and hygiene.   I. Barrick, Ann Louise.   II. Series.
   [DNLM: 1. Geriatric Nursing–methods.   2. Aged.   3. Baths–methods.   4. Dementia–
nursing.   5. Homes for the Aged.   6. Nursing Homes.   7. Patient-Centered Care–methods.
WY 152 B331 2007]
   RC521.B38 2007
   362.1′9683–dc22
                       2007051940

Printed in the United States of America by Bang Printing.

*This book is dedicated to all the direct care workers
who care deeply and struggle daily to provide
compassionate and skillful individualized care.*

Contents

Part II: Special Concerns

Part III: Supporting Caregiving Activities

Contributors

Margaret P. Calkins, PhD
President
I.D.E.A.S., Inc.
Kirtland, Ohio

Johannah Uriri Glover, PhD, MNSc, MSCR, RNP
Assistant Professor
Arizona State University
College of Nursing and Health Innovation
Phoenix, Arizona

Kimberly Horton Hoffman, BSMT (ASCP), CIC
Clinical Manager
Microbiology and Molecular Diagnostics
University of Arkansas for Medical Sciences
Little Rock, Arkansas

Mary Lavelle, MS, RN
Portland, Oregon

Darlene McKenzie, PhD, RN
Professor Emeritus
Oregon Health Sciences University
Portland, Oregon

Lois Miller, PhD, RN
Professor
School of Nursing
Oregon Health Sciences University
Portland, Oregon

Madeline Mitchell, MURP
Project Director (NC)
Data Collection/Management
Cecil G. Sheps Center for Health Services Research
University of North Carolina-Chapel Hill
Chapel Hill, North Carolina

Carla Gene Rapp, PhD, RN, CRRN
Assistant Professor
Duke University School of Nursing
Durham, North Carolina

Joyce H. Rasin, PhD, RN
Associate Professor
Coordinator, Community-Based Nursing
School of Nursing
Widener University
Chester, Pennsylvania

Theresa H. Raudsepp, MSPT
Physical Therapist
Providence Benedictine Nursing Center
Mount Angel, Oregon

LouAnn Rondorf-Klym, PhD, RN, CNS
Senior Clinical Science Manager
Abbott Laboratories, Cardiovascular Medicine
Wilsonville, Oregon

Adele Mattinat Spegman, PhD, RN
Director
Center for Health Research
Geisinger Health System
Danville, Pennsylvania

Karen Amann Talerico, PhD, RN, CNS
President
Amann Talerico Consulting
Portland, Oregon

Jennifer Wood, LPTA, CIMT
Physical Therapy Assistant
In Touch Physical Therapy
Tigard, Oregon

Preface

INTRODUCTION

The purpose of this book is to change current bathing practices that create unnecessary distress and discomfort for persons with dementia. For many persons, bathing remains a pleasant experience. But in some cases, bathing becomes a battle for the care recipient and the caregiver. In the last decade we have learned much about ways to improve care for persons with dementia. We have changed many long held practices and beliefs about what constitutes good care. Yet, many of our standards related to bathing frail elders, particularly those with dementia, remain unchallenged. We hope to change some of your ideas about assisting persons with dementia with bathing by sharing lessons we have learned from many years of clinical practice and 9 years of conducting research in this area.

THE HISTORY OF OUR APPROACH

The approach to understanding and reducing the distress of bathing persons with dementia presented in this book was developed by two multidisciplinary teams of health care providers and researchers: one at Oregon Health Sciences University (OHSU), the second at the University of North Carolina-Chapel Hill (UNC-CH) and John Umstead Hospital (JUH), Butner, North Carolina. During the course of our studies, we have given over 1,000 baths and have worked with more than 50 nursing assistants.

We began at UNC-CH and JUH in 1992 with a grant funded by the National Institute of Aging (NIA) as part of a jointly sponsored initiative with the National Institute of Nursing Research (NINR). We found that there were some nursing assistants who seemed to be able to gain the cooperation of patients who were usually aggressive. We watched what they did and talked with them about their approach to care.

From these experiences we learned much about what helps and what makes the bathing experience worse. We had hoped to be able to develop prescriptions for coping with behavioral symptoms such as yelling and hitting, but we found that we needed a person-centered, psychosocial, problem-solving approach. This enabled us to tailor each bath to the individual. We tried this approach in two nursing homes and found that we could make most bathing experiences more pleasant. We also found that a bed bath seemed to be more comfortable than a shower or tub bath for the most severely impaired individuals. Having the flexibility to bathe a person in a number of different ways was crucial. However, we knew that we would have to test our ideas in a more rigorous study before we could convince others that a shower or tub bath wasn't the only way to get a person clean.

At the same time, the OHSU team was funded by NIA as part of the same joint initiative with NINR to conduct a pilot and feasibility study for a clinical trial on changing nursing home staff's approaches to bathing persons with dementia. Our first aim was to gain a better understanding of how much of a problem aggressive behavior was during bathing residents with dementia (e.g., what kinds of behavioral symptoms occurred and how frequently). Our second aim was to determine if a bedside model of consultation between the direct care provider and a clinical nurse specialist, focused on problem solving and individualizing care, would be effective. We found, as did the UNC team, that when we individualized the bath and the bathing care plan we were able to dramatically reduce the aggressive behaviors.

An important insight we gained was that the relationship between the caregiver and care recipient was essential. Nursing assistants who were able to shift from a task-focused to a person-focused approach were more successful in trying new approaches. Another insight was that nursing assistants valued the support they experienced from the consultant for trying new ideas. They expressed that this was often missing from their coworkers or supervisors. Another important "discovery" was that an in-bed bath, where the person is fully covered with a towel moistened with no-rinse soap and washed and massaged through the towel, often was comforting and soothing for persons who found even an person-directed approach to the shower or tub bath distressing. It was also effective in reducing aggressive behaviors and distress. The nursing assistants who participated also found bathing persons with dementia to be a more positive experience.

Our two teams met because of our mutual interests and decided to join forces in 1995. We believed that our combined approaches from different discipline perspectives (e.g., nursing, medicine, psychology) and the research methods we developed in our first studies would strengthen a larger-scale study across multiple sites. We received funding from the National Institute of Nursing Research to examine two kinds of bathing: a shower and in-room bathing in 15 nursing homes in Oregon and North Carolina. Two of the authors (Joanne Rader, Ann Louise Barrick) worked side by side with the nursing assistants to learn how to increase pleasure and how to decrease distress for the residents included in the study.

Since the completion of our research we have continued to work closely with persons with dementia and their caregivers to increase our knowledge and improve the bathing experience. We have learned that "person-directed" is a better description of our approach. It emphasizes choice and puts the person receiving care first. It also supports caregivers in the provision of care that honors the preferences of the care recipient.

ABOUT THE BOOK

Out of these experiences we developed the approach to bathing persons with dementia discussed in this book.

Part I explores bathing from an overall perspective. The model that guides our work is described in chapter 1. Chapter 2, the history of bathing, illustrates that bathing practices have changed over the years and that there is more than one way to get someone clean. Chapter 3 includes general techniques that help most persons feel more comfortable during bathing. Chapters 4 and 5 cover assessment and interventions for making your bathing plans person-directed. Both are filled with the many ideas gathered while working with very creative and caring nursing assistants. Part II of the book has been updated and is devoted to special concerns related to bathing such as pain, skin care, determining the appropriate level of assistance, transfers, and the environment. An enhanced Part III addresses ways to support caregivers by increasing their understanding of the care recipient's needs and their knowledge of interventions to improve care and comfort. It also emphasizes self-care and system-level changes to promote person-directed care. Several chapters include specific insights and wisdom from direct caregivers.

We worked in health care facilities, but many of the ideas in this book also apply to persons being cared for at home and other settings such as day care programs. Also, although we have focused our discussion on persons with dementia, we believe that many of the approaches discussed in this book are equally useful when caring for other frail elders. Finally, we believe our person-directed problem-solving approach and techniques can be useful during other caregiving activities such as morning and evening care.

Our work is not finished. We invite you to use the model and the solutions we found helpful in your own work. Use your creativity to find the best way to bathe each person in your care. There is no right way to bathe a person, but there are many better ways than the current common practices. Bathing can occur without a battle. We hope you will agree.

We hope that one day nursing homes will offer therapeutic water treatments in relaxing environments. Perhaps some will even be included in *Fodor's Healthy Escapes*. Preposterous? Let's hope not.

Acknowledgments

The authors would like to acknowledge the many people who contributed to this book. The research project, Clinical Trial of Two Bathing Interventions in Dementia, on which this book is based, was funded by National Institute of Nursing Research (NINR) (R01 NR 04188). We are grateful to NINR for recognizing the importance of this work. The authors thank the members of the interdisciplinary Bathing Project Research Team in Oregon and North Carolina. These include: Darlene A. McKenzie and Joyce H. Rasin (coinvestigators); Barbara Stewart (psychometrician) and Gary Koch (biostatistician); C. Madeline Mitchell, LouAnn M. Rondorf-Klym, and Adele Mattinat Spegman (project directors); Charlene Riedel-Leo, Wilaipun Somboontanont, Karen Amann Talerico, Johannah Uriri, and Virapun Wirojratana (team members and graduate research assistants). The authors also thank our consultants: Cornelia Beck, Joyce Colling, Maggie Donius, J.P. Kilborn, and Lynne Morrison. We also wish to acknowledge the School of Nursing, Oregon Health Sciences University (including Diane Berks, administrative assistant), Sheps Center for Health Services Research, University of North Carolina at Chapel Hill, and John Umstead Hospital for resources supporting the project.

The following direct caregivers gave generously of their time and efforts to create and share many of the ideas found in the book: Sandra Boedigheimer, Ruth Burt, Laurie Christopherson, Deb Corwin, Edith S. Durham, Kim Francia, Katrina Hardison, Jose Hernandez, Kathy House, Brenda Jantz, Mineko Leavenworth, Debbie Medina, Angell T. Neal, Beth Parker, Lona Pavao, Rosa Stephens, Rhonda C. Walton, and Janice White. A special thank you goes to all the facilities, families, residents, and staff who assisted with the project. Without their cooperation and assistance none of this would have been possible.

PART I

The Basics

CHAPTER 1

Understanding the Battle

Beverly Hoeffer, Joanne Rader,
Ann Louise Barrick

Imagine yourself as an older person living in a nursing facility or at home with a professional or family caregiver. You grew up when personal care was done in private and seldom discussed. Before you became ill, you bathed in a tub in a small warm bathroom that you decorated to your liking many years ago. However, you are having increasing trouble caring for yourself at home because of memory problems, arthritis, and poor balance. Or perhaps, after falling and bruising yourself badly, you were admitted to a nursing home after a short hospital stay. Today you are confused and have difficulty remembering where you are or recognizing the people who come into your room. You ache from arthritis in your joints and experience pain when you move your arms and legs. You are lying in bed, lost in your memories, when suddenly someone tells you it is time for your shower. You can't figure out who this person is, but before you know it you are swung through the air in a lift and plunked down on a cold chair that looks like a rolling toilet seat. You cry out because you hurt, but the stranger doesn't seem to notice. Instead, she says, "This won't take long." Then she strips off your bedclothes, puts a blanket around your shoulders, and pulls you backward down the hall in the chair. You feel exposed as cold air hits your bottom and thighs. You are afraid and feel that you have no control over what is happening. Your eyes show your anxiety, and you call out, "Help me, help me!" repeatedly, louder and louder. The stranger responds, saying, "I'm just taking you to the shower; I'm not going to hurt you," but it doesn't feel that way to you. Then you are in a small room sitting in this toilet seat chair, stripped naked again. The stranger is spraying you with water, asking you, "Is it too hot?" . . . and you cry out, "Too hot, too hot!" And then, "Oh, I'm cold, I'm cold!" Instead of responding to your cries she raises your arm up. This hurts, and you yell, "No, no, no, no, no, no!" and try to push her away. She tells you she is just washing off the soap, but you feel assaulted and ignored. You don't want a shower; you don't want someone touching you. You . . . just . . . want . . . out . . . of . . . that . . . room and away from the spraying water!

Now, imagine that you are the caregiver trying to help this person take a shower. Bathing is one of the tasks you are assigned, and you want to do a good job. You like taking care of older people, and the last thing you want to do is cause this person pain or distress. But nothing you say or do seems to help. You steel yourself against her cries and complaints of pain and try to ignore them. Afterward, you are upset with the resident for making you feel so incompetent. You no longer look forward to caring for her because it feels like such a battle. You pray that she gets assigned to someone else.

BEHAVIORAL CHANGES IN DEMENTIA

The scenario you just imagined describes an all-too-frequent experience of older persons with dementia and caregivers assigned to help with their personal care. With some alterations in the scenario, it could represent the experience of family caregivers when persons with dementia no longer recognize familiar faces, as can happen in later stages of the illness.

Dementia is not a disease per se but a general term for disorders in which damage to brain cells results in irreversible cognitive decline. To be called dementia, a disorder must have the following features:

- decline in at least two of four essential areas of cognitive functioning (i.e., memory; ability to generate coherent speech or to understand written or spoken language; capacity to plan and make sound judgments; ability to process and interpret visual information)

- impairment in daily functioning, that is, difficulty carrying out daily activities such as shopping or bathing.

Specific brain abnormalities are found in different types of dementia. For example, deposits of protein called plaques and twisted strands of protein called tangles are hallmarks of Alzheimer's disease (AD), the most common dementia. Blocked small arteries and reduced blood flow to areas of the brain due to strokes characterize vascular dementia, the second most common type of dementia. The abnormalities in the central nervous system remain invisible to us, revealed only through autopsies and brain imaging using magnetic resonance imaging (MRI) or computerized axial tomography (CAT) scans (Alzheimer's Association, 2007).

What we as caregivers observe—especially as the dementia progresses—are changes in behavior and communication caused by brain disease. From the caregiver's perspective, behavioral symptoms such as physical and verbal aggression or wandering are frequently viewed as "defiant behaviors," "problematic" or "troublesome" behavior, or "disruptive behaviors." Often this perspective implies that the person with dementia is the problem or is having a problem that needs to be managed. If we turn the lens around and look at behavioral symptoms from the view of the person receiving care, a much different perspective emerges. Behavioral symptoms become ways of communicating experiences such as:

- fear, pain, or distress
- expressions of unmet or unidentified needs
- self-protective behavior against an invasion of personal space or feeling assaulted.

Ultimately, behavior becomes the primary means of communication for persons with dementia when they can no longer express their feelings, needs, or desires verbally or engage in problem solving with others (Algase et al., 1996; Kovach, Noonan, Schlidt, & Wells, 2005).

As the population ages, dementia is becoming an increasingly significant health problem likely to touch all of our lives in some way. AD affects more than 5 million Americans, 96% of whom are 65 and older (Alzheimer's Association, 2007). The prevalence of AD increases with age and, in fact, doubles every 5 years

beyond age 65 (National Institute of Neurological Disorders and Stroke, 2007). Currently, 13% of persons age 65 and over have AD; however, nearly half of persons age 85 and over have AD (Alzheimer's Association, 2007).

The majority of persons with AD are cared for at home, although many families turn to facilities to provide the 24-hour care required in the later stages of this progressive illness. Approximately 70% of all nursing home residents and more than 50% of persons living in assisted living facilities have documented evidence of cognitive impairment or dementia (Alzheimer's Association, 2007). Declining ability to carry out activities of daily living (ADLs) and increasing occurrence of behavioral symptoms during assistance with personal care are often factors that lead to nursing home placement.

PREVALENCE OF BEHAVIORAL SYMPTOMS DURING BATHING

We know that behavioral symptoms of dementia that occur when assisting persons with personal care activities such as bathing are among the most troublesome and difficult for caregivers. Family members surveyed in one study reported that 65% of the persons with dementia they had cared for at home had become aggressive during caregiving (Ryden, 1988). In another study, family members reported that as cognitive impairment became more severe the number of persons with behavioral symptoms increased (Teri, Larson, & Reifler, 1988). They also indicated that assisting with hygiene precipitated the most problematic behaviors. Within nursing homes, behavioral symptoms ranged from an average prevalence of 43% among all persons across a number of studies (Beck, Rossby, & Baldwin, 1991; Beck et al., 1998) to 86% of persons with dementia in one study (Ryden, Bossenmaier, & McLachlan, 1991). In the latter study, nearly three-fourths (72.3%) of aggressive behavior among 124 nursing home residents occurred during caregiving activities involving touch or invasion of personal space.

When caregivers are asked about behavioral symptoms that occur during assistance with personal care such as bathing, they describe behaviors that fall into three general categories. These include:

- resistive behaviors (e.g., pulling away to avoid being bathed; trying to leave bathing area)

- vocal agitation or distress (e.g., crying, loud exclamations such as "Oh! Oh!")
- verbal and physical aggression (e.g., cursing, threatening, hitting, biting, grabbing, pushing).

Study teams in Oregon and North Carolina conducted two surveys to better describe behavioral symptoms that occur during bathing and to better describe the extent to which bathing persons with dementia is difficult for caregivers in nursing facilities. In Oregon, the team collected in-depth data on all residents in one nursing home over a 6-week period (Hoeffer, Rader, McKenzie, Lavelle, & Stewart, 1997). Most residents were bathed weekly in this facility. At the beginning of the survey, 93 of the 102 long-stay residents (91%) required assistance with bathing. Eighty-six of these residents remained in the facility throughout the 6-week period and were included in the study. The nursing assistants who helped residents with bathing completed a checklist of physical, verbal, and sexually aggressive behaviors. The team analyzed data from the first four baths for each resident. Nearly half (41%) were aggressive during at least one of the four baths, and a significant number (16%) were aggressive almost every time (i.e., during three of the four baths). The majority of residents (60%) who were aggressive during one bath had a dementia diagnosis, and an even higher percentage (72%) who were aggressive during almost every bath had a dementia diagnosis. Most of these residents (63%) were both physically and verbally aggressive during bathing while very few were sexually aggressive. By far the most frequent types of physically aggressive behaviors reported by nursing assistants in descending order of frequency were:

- hitting, punching, or slapping
- pinching or squeezing
- pushing or shoving.

Verbally aggressive behaviors reported were fairly evenly distributed among:

- hostile language
- name-calling
- cursing or obscene language.

Aggressive behavior occurred most often during the bath itself but also during undressing and transportation to the bath. The nursing assistants reported other kinds of behaviors not included on the checklist that they found troublesome. These included vocal agitation such as:

- crying
- calling out
- yelling.

The bathing study team in North Carolina took a different approach to learning more about the extent of the problem. The team conducted a survey of 60 nursing homes in North Carolina, drawn randomly from a list of licensed facilities in the state, and of 54 facilities nationwide operated by one proprietary group (Sloane et al., 1995). A questionnaire was mailed to the director of nursing or charge nurse familiar with bathing-related issues in each facility. Seventy-one facilities (62%) completed and returned the questionnaires. Half of these facilities had special care units for persons with Alzheimer's disease.

More than three-fourths of residents usually received a shower that was almost always given in a common bathing area. Very few received a bed bath in their own room. Only half of the nurses reported that they were satisfied with the bathing process in their facility. On average 20% of the residents were reported to be difficult to bathe. Of the residents who were reported to be difficult to bathe, 81% had a diagnosis of dementia. The kinds of behaviors reported as common among persons with dementia who were difficult to bathe were similar to those reported by the caregivers in the Oregon survey. Behaviors reported at least half of the time included physically and verbally aggressive behaviors, resistive behaviors, and vocal agitation.

We know less about the prevalence of behavioral symptoms when family members assist persons with dementia during bathing. In a national telephone survey, 35% of caregivers caring for persons with dementia at home reported that they helped bathe or shower (Alzheimer's Association and National Alliance for Caregiving, 2004). One study of 64 family caregivers of persons with dementia found that 41% assisted their family member during bathing. About half of these found it to be "pretty hard" or "somewhat hard" (Archbold et al., 1997).

WHEN DOES THE BATTLE BEGIN?

We often think of bathing as the time a person spends in the bath or shower. But in caregiving situations, bathing begins with the invitation to the bath. The invitation to the bath is a pivotal time for the battle to start or be prevented. Bathing-related activities during which the battle can occur or be prevented include:

- undressing and dressing
- transfer between the bed or bathtub and a chair
- transportation to the bath or shower room
- bath or shower procedures, including washing
- drying
- hair washing or shaving.

It is not the activity itself that causes behavioral symptoms but the person's experience of the situation from invitation to completion of the bath. The most frequent antecedents or causes of behavioral symptoms during personal care activities such as bathing reported in the literature include:

- touch or invasion of personal space
- perceived loss of control or choice
- anticipation or experience of pain
- feeling that one's needs and preferences are being ignored
- frustration because of declining self-care abilities
- impaired ability to express or communicate needs or feelings
- impaired ability to recognize caregiver's actions as helpful
- tense caregiver appearance, nonengaged communication, or task-oriented behavior.

Because persons with dementia may no longer recognize the caregiver's actions as helpful, they may feel threatened by the invitation to the bath and perceive the bath as an assault. Resistive and aggressive behaviors can be viewed as a defensive response to a perceived threat (Bridges-Parlet, Knopman, & Thompson, 1994) or as protective behavior (Talerico & Evans, 2000), a way for persons to fight back in an attempt to prevent harm from occurring to them during bathing.

A useful way to think about the battle is to view it as a conflict between the agenda of the caregiver and the agenda of the person with dementia. In an observational study of 33 persons with dementia, Kovach and Meyer-Arnold (1996, 1997) found that 92% became agitated or resistive as soon as they were told it was time for a bath. The high prevalence of behavioral symptoms during the invitation to the bath suggests conflicting agendas *from the beginning* between the person with dementia and the caregiver. The caregiver feels that he must give the bath, and the person with dementia, who does not want the bath, feels little control over the situation. Both cope with their conflicting agendas through verbal and nonverbal strategies, all of which have meaning within the context of the bathing situation. Persons with dementia cope with loss of control through behaviors that reflect attempts to resign, share or attain control, and/or regain inner control. Behavioral symptoms (resistive behaviors, vocal agitation, and physical and verbal aggression) occur most often during attempts to attain control or to regain inner control.

Kovach and Meyer-Arnold (1996, 1997) also found caregivers' communication styles and actions related to the occurrence of either calm or agitated behavior among the persons being bathed. Engaged communication included:

- conversation with the person about general topics
- attention to the person's need for comfort and personal preferences during bathing
- reassuring, explaining, and comforting phrases
- diversion
- requests for the person's participation
- humor and compliments.

Nonengaged communication included:

- talking to another caregiver rather than the person
- firm directives and coaxing
- degrading comments and jokes at the person's expense
- saying nothing when the person indicates a desire for communication or shows anxiety.

A person-directed approach—paced to meet the needs of the person being bathed—rather than a task-oriented approach that is often rushed to meet the needs of the caregiver, is key to preventing the battle. It serves to calm and to help the person cope more successfully with the situation.

The physical environment can also contribute to behavioral symptoms during bathing. Environmental factors that lead to discomfort and apprehension, often expressed as resistive, agitated, or aggressive behavioral symptoms, include:

- unfamiliar appearance of bathing rooms in facilities
- bathing apparatus and transportation equipment
- air temperature of the room
- spraying and running water

- unexpected fluctuations in the temperature of the running water
- loud or unusual noises.

Consequently, the battle can be precipitated by events in the physical environment that affect the experience of caregivers and persons with dementia.

Moreover, caregivers report that the support they perceive from their coworkers and supervisors, and from the culture in the facility, influences their approach to bathing persons with dementia. Factors that affect this "caregiving tone" include:

- philosophy
- policy and procedures
- staffing patterns
- structure of day
- equipment and supplies.

The importance of these organizational factors on interactive caregiving is critical. These factors control how much flexibility and caregiving creativity the organization will accept and support. Sometimes caregivers are pressured to conform to rigid policies, procedures, and schedules. Other times, the open, facilitative tone set by the administration gets lost or distorted as it travels to those directly interacting with people with dementia.

Some facilities allow only one towel and one washcloth per bath. This makes it difficult to keep the person covered and warm. Other facilities require showers and do not allow bed baths. In homes, there may be rigid beliefs about how to help someone stay clean or beliefs about when baths can or can't be done. Such policies and beliefs can set the stage for a battle.

Thus, interventions aimed at making bath time a more positive and pleasant experience must take into account the organizational and physical environments that help shape the psychosocial or interpersonal environment in which bathing occurs.

ADDRESSING MYTHS ABOUT BATHING

There are some strongly held beliefs about what is required to keep people clean that need to be addressed. Most of us resist change. It is generally "easier" to do what we have always done. A number of myths about bathing have to be confronted and overcome to champion change related to bathing. Some common myths to consider are:

You Have to Use Lots of Water to Get Clean

Many conscientious caregivers worry that they need to use lots of water in the shower, bath, or bed. However, people maintain cleanliness without the benefit of showers, tubs, or running water at home and in other settings. Washing with attention to detail is more important than how much water you use.

If Caregivers Are Delaying, Deferring, Shortening, or Adapting the Bath or Shower, They Are Trying to Get Out of Work

This is not about being lazy. It may be necessary to create a person-directed plan that meets the person's special needs. Caregivers are still responsible for maintaining the person's hygiene, but they need freedom to adjust the method. Altering the bathing method or schedule actually may reflect the caregiver's commitment to good care and conscientiousness rather than suggest the caregiver is trying to get out of work.

Families Will Insist on a Shower or Tub Bath

Families, like the rest of us, need to be educated. Once presented with the problem (e.g., the person dislikes or fights the bath or shower) and alternative suggestions, families usually understand and agree to try other methods.

There Will Be More Infections and Skin Problems if You Don't Use a Lot of Soap and Water

In our culture, especially during the 20th century, we associated the importance of bathing with the prevention of health problems. However, our experience suggests and data show that modifying the bathing experience and using methods other than the routine bath or shower and plenty of regular soap do not result in more skin problems or infections. A no-rinse soap solution may prevent allergic reactions to soap products and skin problems such as drying.

People Always Feel Better After a Bath or Shower

Just because we feel better after a bath or shower does not mean others do, particularly when it is uncomfortable or they clearly state they don't want it and it is forced upon them. In these cases the person feels distressed or violated.

You Have to Just Go Ahead Because for Most People Who Resist, There Won't Be a "Good" Time

For most people with dementia, developing a plan that keeps them clean and avoids the battle is possible. When the approach, method, day, and time of day are adjusted to the person's needs, bathing without a battle is almost always the outcome.

They Just Forget About the Battle so It Doesn't Matter

Many people who are forced to bathe stay upset for hours following the task. It is almost as if our care plans say, "agitate to the point of aggression one to two times a week during bathing." If the person feels she is being forced or threatened on a regular basis during bathing, our experience suggests that even with memory loss there can be a lasting effect on the person's overall feelings of safety and well-being. Examples of lasting outcomes from forced bathing could include refusal to take medicines, aggressive confrontations with other residents, or further resistance with staff in other care areas.

Regulators, Advocates, and Families Will See It as Possible Neglect

The risk of being misjudged is greater if the only message given is what is not being done, rather than the more positive message of providing person-directed care. The goal is to provide good care by meeting the unique needs of persons with dementia and by avoiding distressing bathing situations. Plans for evaluating problems and for monitoring improvement also need to be presented.

A Person-Directed Approach Will Take More Time, and We Don't Have Time for Extra Care

For most persons, person-directed care can be done in the same amount of time as routine care once you are familiar with new methods, approaches, and techniques. There may be a decrease in overall time spent bathing if you end up bathing some people less frequently.

THE IMPACT OF THE BATTLE

What happens if the battle is not prevented or lessened in some way? What are the consequences for persons with dementia and caregivers? If you have experienced the battle yourself or if you have observed its occurrence at home or in a nursing facility, then the consequences may sound familiar. After experiencing the battle during bathing, persons with dementia may remain upset and agitated throughout the day, which affects their relationships with others with whom they have daily contact. The result is that they may become increasingly isolated and depressed, and others may avoid them. Often they become perceived as difficult and troublesome. Too often the outcome has been the use of physical restraints or the misuse of psychoactive medications to control behavioral symptoms (Talerico & Evans, 2000). We usually think of physical restraints as tying someone down, but other forms of restraint include using several caregivers to hold a person against his will while the bath is given quickly.

Behavioral symptoms, especially aggressive behavior, have serious consequences for caregivers in community and nursing home settings. Caregivers in nursing facilities rate assisting persons with dementia during bathing or showering one of the hardest, if not the hardest, caregiving task that they perform (Miller, 1997; Namazi & Johnson, 1996). Caregivers experience distress and frustration with the caregiving role and may become depressed about their situation. Ultimately, this leads to caregiver burnout and a sense that the burden of caregiving is too great. For family caregivers, the result may be that they can no longer provide the care at home. In nursing facilities, the outcomes are often low staff morale and high staff turnover. Such outcomes are reflected in the findings of a qualitative study conducted in a Dementia Special Care Unit (Miller, 1997). Thirty nursing staff members were interviewed to explore the effects of physically aggressive behavior during hygienic care on them personally and on their practice. Staff reported declines in their physical health, such as pain and exhaustion, and in their mental health. Mental health concerns were:

- concern about their safety during caregiving
- mental exhaustion, frustration, anger, sadness, depression, and anxiety
- fear of being perceived as a poor worker by their peers or administration.

The staff's daily experiences with aggressive behavior during caregiving also resulted in changes in their practice, such as:

- decline in the perceived quality of nursing care
- increase in the potential for staff-to-patient abuse and neglect
- desire to eventually leave the unit, the facility, or the profession.

Findings for this qualitative study are consistent with results from surveys and from anecdotal reports of caregivers' experiences found in the literature.

CONCLUSIONS

For persons with dementia who no longer feel in control of their lives and who are avoided by others, for caregivers who feel burdened and distressed by the experience, and for facilities faced with constant turnover, the costs of the battle are high. The answer lies in challenging the myths and changing the experience for all involved by finding new ways that bathing can occur without a battle.

REFERENCES

Algase, D. L., Beck, C., Kolanowski, A., Whall, A., Berent, S., Richards, K., et al. (1996). Need-driven dementia-compromised behavior: An alternative view of disruptive behavior. *American Journal of Alzheimer's Disease, 11*(6), 10–19.

Alzheimer's Association. (2007). *Alzheimer's disease facts and figures*. Washington, DC: Author (accessible at www.alz.org).

Alzheimer's Association and National Alliance for Caregiving. (2004). *Families care: Alzheimer's caregiving in the United States*. Washington, DC: Alzheimer's Association (accessible at www.alz.org).

Archbold, P., Kaye, J., Keane, T., Lear, J., Miller, F., Parker, N., et al. (1997). [Family caregiving inventory: The caregiver's perspective]. Unpublished data.

Beck, C., Frank, L., Chumbler, N. R., O'Sullivan, P., Vogelpohl, T. S., Rasin, J., et al. (1998). Correlates of disruptive behavior in severely cognitively impaired nursing home residents. *The Gerontologist, 38*(2), 189–198.

Beck, C., Rossby, L., & Baldwin, B. (1991). Correlates of disruptive behavior in cognitively impaired elderly nursing home residents. *Archives of Psychiatric Nursing, 5*(5), 281–291.

Bridges-Parlet, S., Knopman, D., & Thompson, T. (1994). A descriptive study of physically aggressive behavior in dementia by direct observation. *Journal of the American Geriatrics Society, 42*(2), 192–197.

Hoeffer, B., Rader, J., McKenzie, D., Lavelle, M., & Stewart, B. (1997). Reducing aggressive behavior during bathing cognitively impaired nursing home residents. *Journal of Gerontological Nursing, 23*(5), 16–23.

Kovach, C. R., & Meyer-Arnold, E. A. (1996). Coping with conflicting agendas: The bathing experience of cognitively impaired older adults. *Scholarly Inquiry for Nursing Practice: An International Journal, 10*(1), 23–36.

Kovach, C. R., & Meyer-Arnold, E. A. (1997). Preventing agitated behaviors during bath time. *Geriatric Nursing, 18*(3), 112–114.

Kovach, C. R., Noonan, P. E., Schlidt, A. M., & Wells, T. (2005). A model of consequences of need-driven, dementia-compromised behavior. *Journal of Nursing Scholarship, 37*(2), 134–140.

Miller, M. F. (1997). Physically aggressive resident behavior during hygienic care. *Journal of Gerontological Nursing, 23*(5), 24–39.

Namazi, K. H., & Johnson, B. D. (1996). Issues related to behavior and the physical environment: Bathing cognitively impaired patients. *Geriatric Nursing, 17*(5), 234–238; quiz 238–239.

National Institute of Neurological Disorders and Stroke. (2007). *NINDS Alzheimer's disease information page*. Retrieved August 2007, from http://www.ninds.nih.gov/disorders/alzheimersdisease/

Ryden, M. B. (1988). Aggressive behavior in persons with dementia who live in the community. *Alzheimer's Disease and Associated Disorders, 2*(4), 342–355.

Ryden, M. B., Bossenmaier, M., & McLachlan, C. (1991). Aggressive behavior in cognitively impaired nursing home residents. *Research in Nursing & Health, 14*(2), 87–95.

Sloane, P. D., Rader, J., Barrick, A. L., Hoeffer, B., Dwyer, S., McKenzie, D., et al. (1995). Bathing persons with dementia. *Gerontologist, 35*(5), 672–678.

Talerico, K. A., & Evans, L. K. (2000). Making sense of aggressive/protective behaviors in persons with dementia. *Alzheimer's Care Quarterly, 1*(4), 77–88.

Teri, L., Larson, E. B., & Reifler, B. V. (1988). Behavioral disturbance in dementia of the Alzheimer's type. *Journal of the American Geriatrics Society, 36*(1), 1–6.

RESOURCES

Burgener, S. C., Jirovec, M., Murrell, L., & Barton, D. (1992). Caregiver and environmental variables related to difficult behaviors in institutionalized, demented elderly persons. *Journal of Gerontology, 47*(4), P242–P249.

Cohen-Mansfield, J., Marx, M. S., & Rosenthal, A. S. (1990). Dementia and agitation in nursing home residents: How are they related? *Psychology & Aging, 5*(1), 3–8.

Feldt, K. S., Warne, M. A., & Ryden, M. B. (1998). Examining pain in aggressive cognitively impaired older adults. *Journal of Gerontological Nursing, 24*(11), 14–22.

Meddaugh, D. I. (1991). Before aggression erupts. *Geriatric Nursing, 12*(3), 114–116.

Rader, J., Barrick, A. L., Hoeffer, B., Sloane, P. D., McKenzie, D., Talerico, K. A., et al. (2006). The bathing of older adults with dementia. *American Journal of Nursing, 106*(4), 40–49.

Rader, J., Lavelle, M., Hoeffer, B., & McKenzie, D. (1996). Maintaining cleanliness: An individualized approach. *Journal of Gerontological Nursing, 22*(3), 32–38.

Sloane, P. D., Honn, V. J., Dwyer, S. A., Wieselquist, J., Cain, C., & Myers, S. (1995). Bathing the Alzheimer's patient in long-term care: Results and recommendations from three studies. *The American Journal of Alzheimer's Care and Related Disorders*, July/August, 3–11.

CHAPTER 2

Temperatures of the Times: Fluctuations in Bathing Through the Ages

Mary Lavelle

INTRODUCTION

Bathing is an activity of daily living that most Americans take for granted. Many of us count on a shower to wake us up in the morning or look forward to soaking our aches and worries away in a tub at night. It's hard for us to remember that daily bathing is a relatively recent custom even in this country. Along with the availability of water (especially *hot* water), cultural, religious, and social forces determine bathing traditions. Even today, bathing may be seen as a task or chore rather than as a pleasurable activity in areas where obtaining or heating water is difficult. Many elders, both foreign born and native, may not remember bathing with deep fondness. Prior to the introduction of water heaters for private homes, bathwater was often heated on the stove and shared by all of the family members. Stoddard (1996) remembers Saturday night baths in a galvanized tub, from the vantage point of the last bather—the "dark ages when cleanliness, rather than being next to godliness, was next to impossible" (p. 48). As we caregivers go about our daily work, helpful reminders include:

- Beliefs and practices about bathing have changed over time.
- Personal bathing histories can be fascinating, unique to the individual, and helpful to discover.
- Bathing "challenges" have stimulated creativity and humor throughout the ages.

Early Bathing and the Discovery of Vapour

It's not clear how the practice of what we call bathing actually started for early human beings. Wright (1960) surmises that an accidental tumble into a cold river may have led to the discovery of bathing's refreshing effects. However, this chilly invigoration wasn't for everyone— "vapour baths" were invented in Asia thousands of years ago. These "prehistoric" bathers heated river pebbles in wood fire pits in their huts, soaked the hot rocks in water, and enjoyed the steam. The invention spread along four different routes over the centuries and was modified for local conditions. Differences between the Nordic and Arab countries in the use of dry or humid heat continue to this day, and techniques used by North American Indians in sweat lodges can be traced to the "vapour baths" of prehistoric times (De Bonneville, 1998; Zucker, Hummel, & Hogfoss, 1983). The first known bathtub dates back 3,600 years; it came from a palace at Knossos on Crete where the Minoans developed magnificent bathing facilities with intricate artwork (De Bonneville, 1998; Rosen, 1993; Wright, 1960).

Bathing in Ancient Civilizations

In Western civilization, Greek baths were the earliest forms of communal bathing (see Figure 2.1). Early Greek baths were brief, cold, and invigorating until later centuries when hot water and hot air baths became popular. Ancient Egyptian palaces contained bathing rooms and stoves for heating water. Tomb illustrations show servants trickling water from highly decorated vases upon the queen (De Bonneville, 1998; Scott, 1939; Wright, 1960). After the Romans conquered the Mediterranean world, they raised the art of bathing to a height never again achieved. Roman engineers designed aqueducts that brought amazingly large amounts of water over long distances. They also

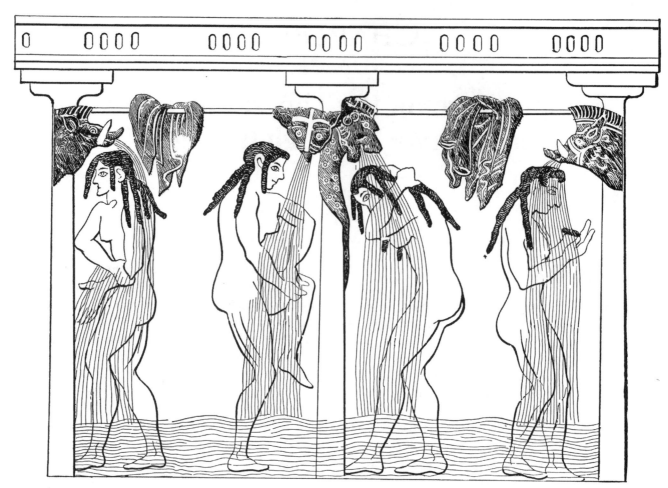

FIGURE 2.1   Greek shower.
Source: **Gerhard (1908), page 155.**

developed methods for heating this water to provide comfort to large crowds. They brought their love of water to the lands they conquered and built colossal thermal baths that became the focus of communal life. The Baths of Caracalla could hold 1,600 bathers at a time. Smaller baths coexisted with these larger public institutions. The Romans believed bathing was therapeutic and that it relieved pain and worry. Health specialists worked out detailed bathing regimens for certain afflictions and conditions. Wine and food were often enjoyed during bathing (Mumford, 1961; Rosen, 1993; Wright, 1960; Yegul, 1995).

The Decline of Bathing With the Decline of Rome

As Christianity developed, it had a tendency to reject Roman values. Christian beliefs about materialism and vanity, along with the baths' reputation for licentious behavior, led to a condemnation of baths by the church at the end of the fourth century (De Bonneville, 1998; McLaughlin, 1971). Invasions, wars, and internal events resulted in the decline of the Greco-Roman world. Baths were gradually abandoned as water supplies were cut off and cities and towns were destroyed (De Bonneville, 1998; Rosen, 1993). Nonetheless, certain types of baths were still allowed, and beliefs about bathing differed among sects. Monasteries were the guardians of culture and sanitation during this time. Benedictine monks, some of the earliest nurses, kept bathing to a minimum but bathed the ill who came to their monasteries for care (Risse, 1999).

Bread, Baths, and Scandalous Behavior

Public baths were resurrected during the medieval period. Bath rituals indicative of festivity and celebration, in addition to hygiene routines, are recorded in wood-cuts. Ideas brought from Asia were adapted in Britain: Steam generated from bread making was used to heat water for "Turkish" baths. Members of the Barbers' Company offered haircuts and shaves to the bathers and also performed medical procedures such as bloodletting and cupping (De Bonneville, 1998; Wright, 1960).

Every Northern European city had bathhouses, and bathing was a family outing that spread to the rural areas. Bathers steamed and sweated at least every other week in the public baths, and, as in Roman times, the act of coming together in the bathhouse promoted sociability without embarrassment about nudity. People chatted and ate food in the bath. Sometimes the focus of the bath was more medicinal when bathers were treated for inflammatory conditions and pains.

Public bathing again gradually fell into disuse for a few hundred years, possibly because of the spread of disease, activities of "loose women" and "lecherous men," or the lack of fuel for heating water. Nudity fell out of favor as well, and people chose to wash just their face and hands in private (De Bonneville, 1998). The spread of the plague and other epidemics in Europe coincided with a growth in the belief that water could penetrate bodies and bring in diseases (Vigarello & Birrell, 1988).

Fever Treatments

Baths continued to be used for medical treatments. A picture from the 17th century illustrates a "fever bag." Water was poured through an outlet near the head and drained into a bucket at the foot of the bed. Whether the water for these treatments was heated or not is unknown, but cold water treatment for fever had been advocated until recently (see Figure 2.2).

River and Sea Bathing: Real and Imagined

In France, swimmers in 1750 began the "unstoppable craze" of river bathing (De Bonneville, 1998, p. 43). Sea bathing began to catch on at that time in England, although some entered the sea in a machine, dragged by horses, which allowed them to stay covered under a hood. Sea bathing was not intended for pleasure or even cleanliness but as a medical treatment for glandular difficulties (McLaughlin, 1971; Wright, 1960). For those far from rivers and seas, a special bathing appliance was invented in the late 1800s that was said to be much adver-

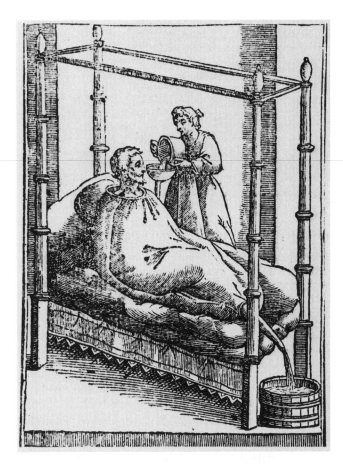

FIGURE 2.2   A 17th-century feverbag.
Source: **Courtesy of the National Library of Medicine History of Medicine collection.**

tised in Europe—the "portable wave bath." The motion of the bather was thought to be more exhilarating than quiet water (Gerhard, 1908, p. 24; see Figure 2.3).

Cold Water and the Revival of Bathing

The Hydropathic Water-Cure Movement or Water-Cure Craze adopted from Europe took hold in the United States in the mid-1800s and began to change Americans' attitudes toward bathing. Hydropathy stressed the benefits of *cold* water, both for drinking and for bodily application, and the benefits of changes in personal habits for prevention and healing. This movement challenged traditional medical treatments such as purging and bloodletting and provided alternative ways of thinking about health, healing, and the role of women in medicine. It emphasized patient participation and offered ideas that may resonate with us in the 21st century, although some

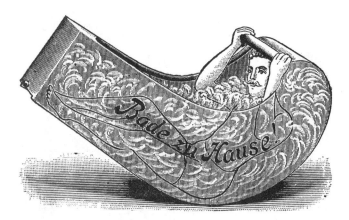

FIGURE 2.3 A portable wave bath.
Source: **Gerhard (1908), page 24.**

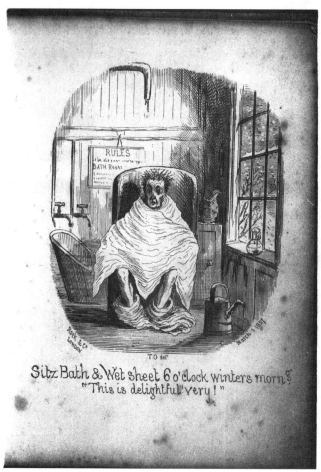

Sitz Bath & Wet sheet 6 o'clock winters morn
"This is delightful very!"

FIGURE 2.4 A sitz bath cartoon from the 19th century.
Source: **Courtesy of the National Library of Medicine, History of Medicine.**

of these applications are rather quirky (Cayleff, 1987; Trall, 1851; Weiss & Kemble, 1967).

Hydropathic physicians prescribed very specific baths for particular health conditions. The humorist Mark Twain, describing his mother's enthusiasm for treatments of the day, reported that she stood him naked in the backyard every morning and threw buckets of cold water on him to see what effect it would have. Then she wrapped him in a cold wet sheet and put him to bed where he would sweat (Ober, 1997). Cartoonists of the day also made fun of these chilly curative treatments (see Figure 2.4).

Bathing for Cleanliness Catches on

A culture of cleanliness began to take off in the later part of the 19th century as ideals associated with gentility and good health became prevalent, and manufacturers of tubs, soap, and plumbing systems caused cleanliness to become a big business (Bushman & Bushman, 1988; Wright, 1960). As municipal water systems were constructed, commercial bathhouses offered middle- and upper-class patrons a variety of baths (Williams, 1991). For Americans moving westward into the frontier, portable equipment for vapour baths was available. Some Americans carried rubber tubs along with them in wagons (Myres, 1991).

Municipal baths were built in Europe to provide for those who moved into crowded cities as part of the Industrial Revolution; in Japan, public baths were well established by the turn of the century (Gerhard, 1908). In the United States, wealthier members of society installed indoor plumbing and built private baths as standards of personal cleanliness changed, but immigrants were crowded into city slums without facilities. A public bath movement developed slowly as part of sanitary movements and Progressive Era reforms. Several summer bathing facilities, so-called floating baths, were developed along rivers and ocean fronts in the first move toward providing facilities for the poor. Cleanliness became important for social and economic mobility. Bath reformers advertised and strenuously brought the "gospel of cleanliness" to the public schools (Armstrong, 1914; Paine, 1905; Quincy, 1900; Smith, 1905; Todd, 1910; Williams, 1991). Figure 2.5, published in 1905, shows how many thought bathing was worth the wait.

The public bath movement reached its peak in the United States in 1910. As homes in neighborhoods near the baths converted to indoor plumbing in the

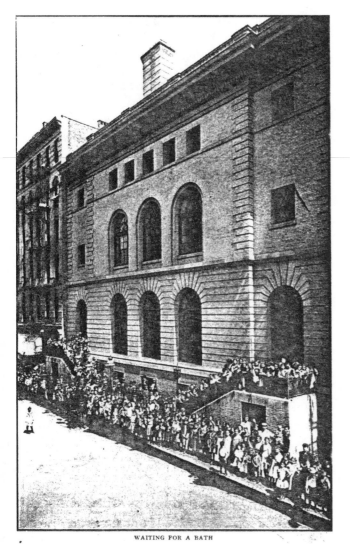

FIGURE 2.5   Lined up for a bath in New York City, 1905.
Source: **Smith (1905), page 566.**

1920s, public bathing declined and bathing facilities became a requirement for low-income housing built during the New Deal. By the beginning of World War II public baths served only a small minority (Williams, 1991).

SUMMARY

Bathing has been viewed as therapeutic at times and dangerous at other times. In ancient Greece and Rome, bathing was pleasurable and hygienic. Elaborate engineering provided water and heat, and bathers could

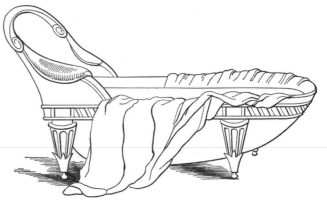

FIGURE 2.6   Sofa bath.
Source: **Gerhard (1908), page 20.**

socialize in pleasant, sometimes artistically decorated, surroundings. Communal bathing was later seen as unhygienic in some periods and as immoral in others. Cold water therapy became popular as an alternative to harsher medical regimens; bathing for fevers was popular for many years. Natural hot springs were viewed as places of healing early on; the popularity of these spas continues to this day.

Perhaps when you think about the effects of bathing you'll be reminded about how the environment and customs determine the experience. Though the air bath, cold water cures, bathing with 1,600 others, and even the portable wave bath have gone out of favor, it's interesting to think about the variety of approaches people have used over time. Perhaps ideas about past and present bath practices will help you transform bathing into pleasurable and comforting spa-like rituals for elders rather than into a cleansing task that just needs to get done (see Figure 2.6).

REFERENCES

Armstrong, D. (1914). Public bath advertising campaign. *The Survey, 31*, 646–647.

Bushman, R. L., & Bushman, C. L. (1988). The early history of cleanliness in America. *The Journal of American History, 74*(4), 1213–1238.

Cayleff, S. (1987). *Wash and be healed: The water-cure movement and women's health.* Philadelphia: Temple University Press.

De Bonneville, F. (1998). *The book of the bath.* New York: Rizzoli.

Gerhard, W. P. (1908). *Modern baths and bath houses.* New York: Wiley.

McLaughlin, T. (1971). *Dirt: A social history as seen through the uses and abuses of dirt.* New York: Stein and Day.

Mumford, L. (1961). *The city in history: Its origins, its transformations, and its prospects.* New York: Harcourt, Brace & World.

Myres, S. L. (1991). *Westering women and the frontier experience, 1800-1915.* Albuquerque: University of New Mexico Press.

Ober, K. P. (1997). The Pre-Flexnerian reports: Mark Twain's criticism of medicine in the United States. *Annals of Internal Medicine, 126*(2), 157–163.

Paine, R. (1905). The bathers of the city. *The Outing Magazine, 46,* 558–569.

Quincy, J. (1900). Municipal progress in Boston. *The Independent, 52,* 424–426.

Risse, G. B. (1999). *Mending bodies, saving souls: A history of hospitals.* New York: Oxford University Press.

Rosen, G. (1993). *A history of public health.* Baltimore: Johns Hopkins University Press.

Scott, G. R. (1939). *The Story of Baths and Bathing.* London: T. Werner Laurie.

Smith, B. H. (1905). The public bath. *The Outlook, 79,* 567–577.

Stoddard, M. G. (1996, July/August). Grime and punishment. *The Saturday Evening Post,* 48–49.

Todd, R. E. (1910). Four new city baths and gymnasiums. *The Survey, 23,* 680–683.

Trall, R. T. (1851). *The hydropathic encyclopedia: A system of hydropathy and hygiene, in eight parts, designed as a guide to families and students, and a text-book for physicians.* New York: Fowler & Wells.

Vigarello, G., & Birrell, J. (1988). *Concepts of cleanliness: Changing attitudes in France since the Middle Ages.* New York: Cambridge University Press.

Weiss, H. B., & Kemble, H. R. (1967). *The great American water-cure craze: A history of hydropathy in the United States.* Trenton, NJ: Past Times.

Williams, M. T. (1991). *Washing "the great unwashed": Public baths in urban America, 1840–1920.* Columbus: Ohio State University Press.

Wright, L. (1960). *Clean and decent: The fascinating history of the bathroom & the water closet, and of sundry habits, fashions & accessories of the toilet, principally in Great Britain, France & America.* New York: Viking.

Yegul, F. K. (1995). *Baths and bathing in classical antiquity.* Cambridge, MA: MIT Press.

Zucker, J., Hummel, K., & Hogfoss, B. (1983). *Oregon Indians: Culture, history and current affairs, an atlas and introduction.* Portland, OR: Western Imprints, Oregon Historical Society.

CHAPTER 3

General Guidelines for Bathing Persons With Dementia

Ann Louise Barrick, Joanne Rader

Bathing can be a particularly sensitive issue for persons with dementia. People with brain disease can become confused easily and will often misinterpret what others are doing or saying. Often even the smallest thing that is unpleasant, such as water in the eyes or ears, can make them respond with fear or violence. These responses are not something the person can control. However, we can control the way we interact with them and provide care activities in a way that minimizes discomfort and fits their personal preferences.

Each person has a set of characteristics, routines, wants, and needs that work for that person and make a good day. The better we know the person, the better and easier the care. Person-directed care puts the person first instead of putting the policies and procedures of the facility and routines of the home first. Person-directed care strives to support the choices of the person being assisted and to involve that person in as much decision making as possible. This focused care recognizes the inherent value of each individual and is focused on supporting strengths and abilities, capacity for social contribution, unique values, and preferences and living habits. This method of care also focuses on promoting autonomy and choice.

Person-directed care also recognizes that some individuals lack cognitive abilities to tell us with words what their wishes are. However, their past choices and present behavior give us key information about what will most honor their wishes in the current situation. In these cases, family members and direct caregivers who work with them on a daily basis need to have the ability to adapt routines to fit the person's expressed and implied

wishes. For example, a person who is physically resisting at the entrance of the bathroom may be telling us that we need to find another way to wash him, that we need to encourage and support him, or that the current way is too frightening, painful, or overwhelming. Therefore, we should not place on his care plan, "shower twice a week." Instead, we should say: "dislikes the shower, bathe in his room, on the bed, keeping him covered and warm. If the person resists this also, come back later. If his preferred, consistent caregiver is off on bath day, consider postponing the bath." Table 3.1 illustrates how care planning is different when it is person-directed rather than institutionally focused.

Here are some general guidelines to help you create person-directed bathing. These strategies apply to every individual and bath.

- *Focus more on the person than on the task.* Meeting individual preferences and emphasizing the well-being of the person being bathed is more important than providing care in an efficient manner. The "car-wash approach" (see Figure 3.1) may get the person clean, but the cost to both you and the other person is high. Observe the person's feelings and reactions (Is there fear/pain?). Always protect privacy and dignity.
- *Be flexible.* Modify your approach to meet the needs of the person. This involves adapting (a) your methods (e.g., distracting the person with singing while bathing), (b) the physical environment (e.g., choosing correct size of shower chair), and (c) the procedure (e.g., dividing up tasks such as hair washing and bathing).
- *Use persuasion, not coercion.* Help the person feel in control. Give choices and respond to individual requests. Support remaining abilities. Negotiate or

We would like to acknowledge Debbie Medina, our coauthor on the previous version of this chapter.

TABLE 3.1   Traditional vs. Person-Directed Planning

Traditional Planning	Person-Directed Planning
Planning **FOR** the person	Planning **WITH** the person
Talking **ABOUT** the person	Talking **WITH** the person
Starting with what's **"WRONG"** with the person	Starting with what is **IMPORTANT** to the person
HEALTH and **SAFETY** dictate care	Health and safety are addressed in context of the person's **WISHES** and **CHOICES**
OTHERS are "in charge"	Power is **SHARED**

find a reason that the person can accept. The goal is for you to help the person get to "yes." Use shortcuts such as no-rinse soap. Use distractions such as food or conversation when necessary to help the person feel more pleasure. Use a supportive, calm approach, and praise the person often.

- *Be prepared.* Gather everything you will need for the bath before approaching the person. Where will the bath take place? In the person's room? In the bathroom? Warm the room. What special products will you need? Do you have enough towels? Washcloths? If the person likes to be dressed in the bathroom, do you have all of the person's clothes?

- *Stop.* When a person becomes distressed, stop and assess the situation. It is not "normal" for a person to cry, moan, or fight during bathing. Look for the underlying reason for the behavior. What can you do to prevent the person from becoming more upset?

- *Ask for help.* Talking with others about ways to meet the needs of the person gives you an opportunity to find different ways to help make the bath more comfortable.

GENERAL STRATEGIES FOR STOPPING THE BATTLE

Simple interventions can often be surprisingly effective in reducing the stress of the bathing experience for you and the person you are bathing. These can be divided into five areas:

- Meet personal needs.
- Adapt your interpersonal/relationship approach.
- Adapt the physical environment.
- Adapt the organizational environment.
- Stop the battle.

Meeting Personal Needs

The most common personal needs expressed by elders during bathing are freedom from pain, cold, and fear, and a wish for a sense of control over what happens to them. Strategies for addressing the needs of most elderly people include:

- Cover! Cover! Cover! Keep the person covered as much as possible or desired to keep them warm and minimize muscle tension (see Figures 3.2 and 3.3). Wash one area at a time and then cover the area.
- Time the bath to fit the person's history, preferences, and mood.
- Bathe a person before she is dressed for the day to eliminate extra movement and discomfort.
- Move slowly and prepare the person prior to moving him/her by counting or giving a warning.

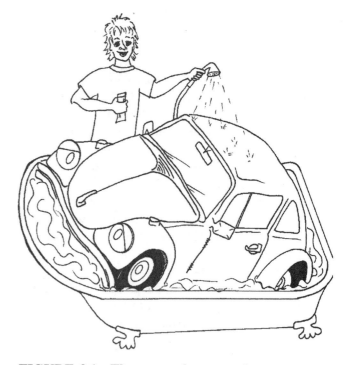

FIGURE 3.1   The car wash approach.

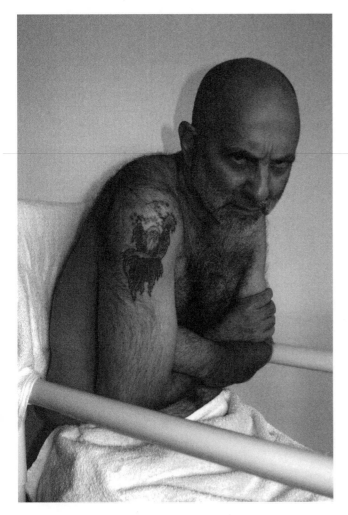

FIGURE 3.2   Person wet and cold.

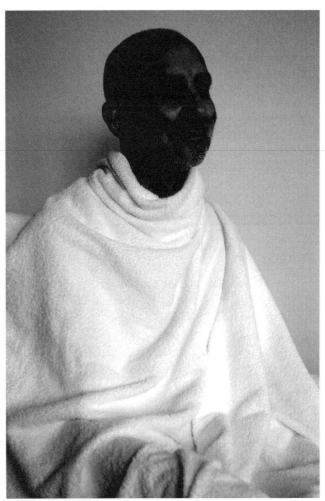

FIGURE 3.3   Person covered and warm.

- Watch out for legs and other body parts that might get bumped or injured when moving.
- Minimize the number of moves during the bath.
- Evaluate the need for medical treatments for pain control.
- Start with the least sensitive area so that pain and tension do not immediately escalate. Wash the most sensitive area (as defined by the person being bathed) last.
- Ask the person who is able to talk what will help her feel better.
- Use soft cloths such as baby washcloths on sensitive skin.
- Use a gentle touch.
- Pat dry rather than rub to decrease discomfort.

- Use another method for bathing if the person is fearful of tubs with mechanical lifts.

Adapting Your Interpersonal/ Relationship Approach

The relationship between you and the person you are bathing is enhanced by the following general approaches:

- Address the person by his/her preferred name.
- Encourage self-care if appropriate.
- Engage the person in conversation (e.g., talk about things, events, and persons of interest to the person; ask the person's opinion).
- Give compliments and praise.

- Tell the person what you are doing at all times and avoid surprises.

Caregiver Wisdom

You have to try to get the person to trust you. The relationship is really important. Sit and talk with the person. Know what their needs are. If you tell someone you are going to do something, always do it. Everyone needs a friendly face and a kind word.

Ruth Burt, CNA, Oxford Manor, Oxford, NC

- Adjust your language to match the person's ability to understand (see chapter 6). Use verbal interventions with persons who can still talk, and pay special attention to nonverbal behaviors with persons who cannot talk.
- Follow the person's lead. Talk if the person responds and is not overwhelmed. Sing if the person likes it. Be silent if that works best. Too much talking can increase agitation in some people.
- Avoid the word "bath" with persons who do not like to bathe. Use an expression that is acceptable (e.g., wash up, spit bath).
- Speak calmly, slowly, and simply while facing the person.
- Apologize repeatedly at any sign of distress.
- Go slow, giving the person enough time to process your questions and requests.
- Provide gentle, reassuring touch if tolerated and desired.
- Use distractions such as objects to hold, candy, or other food that the person likes to help soothe the person and give her something else to do. Use caution in offering food. Check for dietary and swallowing restrictions first.
- Let the person know what is left to do (e.g., "I'll wash your back, and then we are done").

Adapting the Physical Environment

The temperature of the bathing room, the design and comfort of the shower chair, lighting, noise, and sense of privacy all affect the person's bathing experience. Try the following suggestions to modify the physical environment and to make the bath more pleasant:

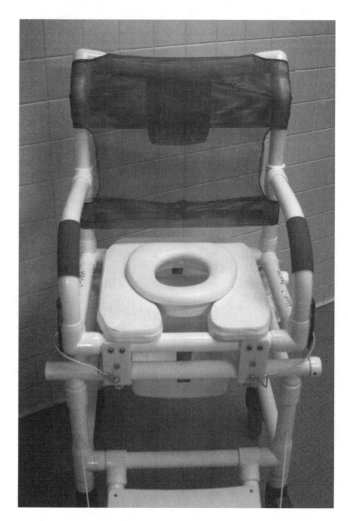

FIGURE 3.4   Shower chair with padded insert.

- Pad the shower chair to increase comfort (see Figure 3.4). Padded shower chairs can be purchased. You can also use a padded child's toilet seat insert or washcloths around the edge of the seat to increase comfort.
- In the tub use a shower bench covered with a towel, because it is often very difficult for someone who has dementia or who is stiff or frail to sit down in the tub.
- Turn the heat on or run the hot water in the bathroom prior to giving a bath to give the room time to warm up.
- Adapt the equipment so it fits the person. For example, for a small person, use a short shower chair or stool with a standard chair to keep the feet from dangling and to promote a feeling of security and safety.

- Use beds that can be raised or lowered as needed for staff and resident safety and for comfort during transfers.
- Reduce annoying noise levels.
- Provide soothing music if the person seems to enjoy it.
- Try adding positive aromas such as potpourri or scented oil.

Adapting the Organizational Environment

Rigid policies and practices related to frequency and types of bathing will hamper your ability to provide person-directed care. Some possible ways to modify the organizational environment include:

- Use consistent assignment of caregivers so there is an opportunity to get to know the person and to establish a relationship.
- Encourage flexibility in bath schedules. If a person prefers a bath in the evening, arrange to have it done then.
- Use two care providers if needed (e.g., one to wash, one to engage in conversation or to distract with food).
- Try a different kind of bath (e.g., bed bath, chair bath) if a tub bath or shower causes distress.
- Invite family members to give input or to help with the bath.
- Respect the person's right to say "no."

Stopping the Bath

When you are caring for someone with dementia, it is frustrating when your kindest, best efforts result in your being yelled at and kicked. The person may misinterpret what you are saying and quickly become angry. She may say one thing and mean another. There are day-to-day, and sometimes moment-to-moment, changes in thinking and behavior. The person may say that she understands what you are asking and then may fail to do it. These are just some of the many puzzling situations you are likely to face. Knowing what to do when these things happen and knowing when to stop the bath are important.

As mentioned earlier, it should not be considered standard or normal to have screams, cries, and protests coming from the bathing room. Bathing battles have the potential to be physically and emotionally harmful to both parties. When signs of distress occur during a bath follow these steps:

1. Stop what you are doing.
2. Assess for causes of distress.
3. Adjust your approach.
4. Evaluate the effectiveness of the new approach.
5. Shorten or stop the bath.
6. Try to end on a positive note before you leave.
7. Reapproach later if necessary to finish washing critical areas.

If you are unable to calm the person and make the bath more comfortable, you will need to shorten the bath. If the person is very aggressive, you will need to stop the bath. Wash only what is necessary for good health. If the person becomes so distressed that you must end the bath, try to end with something pleasant, such as offering a cup of coffee or a backrub. This may make it easier when you return. The next two chapters contain ideas to use when these general strategies do not reduce the stress of the bath.

NOTE

The material in this chapter was adapted with permission from: Rader, J., & Barrick, A. L. (2000). Ways that work: Bathing without a battle. *Alzheimer's Care Quarterly, 1*(4), 35–49.

CHAPTER 4

Assessing Behaviors

Ann Louise Barrick, Joanne Rader, Madeline Mitchell

The general strategies in chapter 3 can help bathing be more pleasant. To get the best results, you need to tailor your care to the specific needs of each person you are assisting. This requires:

- knowing a lot about the person
- having a large number of options handy
- being flexible.

The next two chapters prepare you for this individualized, person-directed approach. This is a continuous process that is useful anytime there is evidence of distress (see Figure 4.1). The steps include:

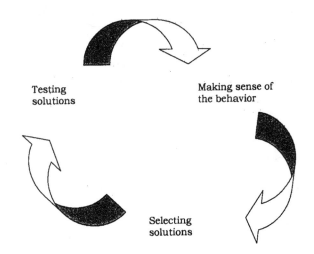

FIGURE 4.1 Steps in the person-directed approach.

Being nice is not enough! We observed many caregivers using a calm, gentle approach. But without understanding why the person was distressed, they were unable to make the bathing experience more pleasant. Understanding the meaning of behavioral symptoms, from the person's perspective, and seeing them as an expression of an unmet need will open up a wide range of person-directed solutions. This approach requires a careful assessment of the person and of the behavior to uncover the trigger(s) or cause(s) of the behavior.

Understanding the Person

Knowing as much as you can about the person will help you understand why the behavior might be occurring as well as help you choose strategies to reduce it. The Personal Information Data Sheet (see chapter appendix) can be used for gathering the following information:

- *Personal history:* What are the person's past accomplishments, topics of interest, family relations, hobbies, likes, and dislikes?
- *Physical health:* Find out the person's remaining abilities as well as problems including mobility limitations, areas of pain, sensitivity to cold, medications, visual and hearing impairments, and diseases. Knowledge of current health problems, such as pain, that may cause behaviors is crucial.
- *Personality factors:* Does the person have a sense of humor? Is she outgoing and gregarious or introverted and quiet? Has a need for control been important?
- *Psychosocial well-being and mood:* Is the person involved and interested in daily activities? Is there any evidence of depression? Do friends and family visit?
- *Preferences for bathing and dressing:* Find out about past bathing habits as well as the current preferred time of day and type of bath. Can the person undress or dress without assistance? The Bathing Preferences and Practices Form (see chapter appendix) can be given to the family to gather this information.

- *Level of dementia:* How does the person communicate? Are there memory impairments, difficulty with attention, impaired judgment, or impulse control?

Sources of this information include:

- the person
- the family
- other caregivers
- other staff (housekeepers, dietary, social services, activities)
- medical/clinical record.

Caregiver Wisdom

One gentleman was verbally gruff with me the first few times I bathed him. But I developed a comfortable, consistent routine for him; he saw that I cared about how he felt. Also, I always explained to him what we were doing. He became very cooperative and pleasant. After the fourth bath, he told his wife I was so good that I needed a raise in pay! That made me feel good. That is a success story.

Debbie Medina, CNA, Hood River
Care Center, Hood River, OR

Describe the Behavior

Work on only one behavior at a time. Although there may be several different behaviors causing concern, choose the one that is most upsetting, such as hitting. Observe the person carefully when the behavior occurs. Gather as much information as you can about this behavior. The Behavior Tracking Log (Exhibit 4.1) can be used to document your observations and answers to the following questions about the behavior:

- What is the person doing that indicates that he is distressed (e.g., crying, yelling, grabbing, trying to hit, trying to leave)?
- When does the behavior occur (e.g., when the water is turned on, during cleansing of the feet)?
- Is this a new behavior?
- Where does the behavior occur (e.g., in the shower room but not the bedroom)?

- Who is involved when this happens?
- How often does this happen?
- What happens just before the behavior?
- What happens after?
- What seems to help?
- What seems to make the behavior worse?
- What makes this behavior a concern?

These questions help you identify behavioral triggers. Triggers may be people, places, or events that cause the behavior to occur or cause it to get worse. Sometimes behaviors have multiple triggers. Refusal to enter the shower room may be triggered by modesty, physical discomfort of a shower chair, or fear of being cold.

Learn to Identify Causes/Triggers of the Behavior

Every behavior has meaning, but often the meaning has to be uncovered or discovered. This may be a difficult process because behaviors are complex and may have many different triggers. You have to figure out what the person is trying to communicate. Try viewing the bath through the eyes, ears, and feelings of the person. For example, think about:

- How you would respond if you thought a stranger was trying to take your clothes off?
- How it would feel to have water that is too hot or too cold hitting you?
- What might help to make you more comfortable?

Look for the cause of the behavior anytime there is a sign of discomfort. Systematic observation is crucial. Identify patterns of behavior and what is happening at those times. For example, the behavior may occur more often in a shower than in a tub bath or when there are two caregivers instead of one. Uncover clues to factors or triggers that might be affecting the behavior. You may need to make a "best guess" about possible causes of behavior because a clear cause may not emerge. When looking for causes of behaviors it is helpful to assess:

- *Personal factors:* individual physical and emotional factors such as pain, cold, physical illness or limitations, level of dementia, fear, or need for control

Exhibit 4.1   Behavior Tracking Log

Behavior Tracking Log

Name: _____   Date: _____

When does it happen? (e.g., when the water is turned on)	
Who is present? (e.g., caregivers, Mary and Jane)	
Where does the behavior occur? (e.g., in the shower but not in the tub)	
What is the person doing? (e.g., hitting, biting)	
What happens before? (e.g., the spray is focused on the person's chest)	
What happens after? (e.g., the caregiver says she'll hurry)	
What makes it better? (e.g., the caregiver apologizes)	
What makes it worst? (e.g., the caregiver ignores the hitting and keeps showering the person)	

- *Relationship factors:* how you relate to the person and his/her unique needs and how the person relates to you
- *Physical environment:* physical features of the bathing environment including room temperature and comfort of equipment
- *Organizational environment:* administrative policies and procedures that impact the caregiver's time, approach, flexibility, creativity, and work routines.

Learn the Personal Needs and Capabilities of the Person You Are Bathing

Personal needs can be expressed both verbally and nonverbally. Common concerns expressed by persons receiving a bath include being in pain, being cold, and feeling a lack of control, anxiety, or fear. Table 4.1 illustrates the many ways these concerns may be expressed.

The most common personal causes of distress are related to physical needs, emotional needs, or dementia-related problems.

Physical needs include:

- *Pain:* It is important to look for sources of unnecessary or excess disability caused by untreated pain. What physical handicaps does the person have? Is she stiff? Does she have contractures (limited range of motion)? Other common causes of pain during bathing include sensitive skin, sensitive feet, stroke-related pain, and arthritis. Refer to chapter 7 for a more detailed discussion of pain.
- *Acute illnesses:* A change in physical health can trigger agitation or aggression. A sudden change in behavior is often the first clue to physical illness in a person who cannot communicate discomfort verbally. Look for other signs of acute illness such as lethargy, agitation, increased temperature, or congestion. Signs of delirium include:

- Difficulty in shifting or in sustaining attention
- Stupor or decreased level of consciousness
- Tactile and/or auditory hallucinations
- Disturbed sleep/wake cycle
- Fluctuations in symptoms.

TABLE 4.1 Different Expressions of Concern During Bathing

	Pain	Feeling Lack of Control	Anxiety/Fear	Cold
Verbal/Vocal	Says: "That hurts" Asks to "stop" Repeatedly asks for help Complains Moans and groans Screams and yells Mutters in a distressed tone Swears Unusual noise he makes intensifies in volume and in pitch Cries	Says: "No!" Threatens, curses, and insults Makes demands Screams and yells Says: "Why are you doing this to me?"	Screams and yells Calls for help from others: a spouse, friend, the police, 911 Calls out in pain before being touched Says: "You're going to kill me"	Says: "I'm cold!" Says: "I'm hot!" Yells and screams
Nonverbal	Winces Grimaces Flinches Rubs area Fidgets, repositions self Generalized tension Pulls away or other avoidance behaviors Extreme facial expressions Restlessness Rocks Rigidity Clenches fist Slow movements Noisy breathing Hits Bites	Pulls away, pushes away Hits Bites or spits Grabs Scowls Scratches Refuses to enter bathroom Points finger at caregiver Attempts to leave	Rigidity Grabs Worried/fearful expression Clenches fist Wrings hands Jittery Shivers Withdraws from caregiver touch	Shivers Tries to cover self Cold hands and feet Trembling lips

- *Cold:* Many individuals become sensitive to cold as they age. It takes longer to warm up once a person is cold. Clues that a person is cold are complaints about the temperature of the room or water, shivering, and efforts to cover up.

Look for Signs of Untreated Pain or Illness

Mrs. Gross cries throughout her bath. Efforts to comfort her or to change her bathing routine do not help. Staff members report that she has recently begun pacing the halls, mumbling in an agitated manner. This mumbling becomes louder and develops into crying when someone tries to help her dress or eat.

<u>Discussion:</u> *Mrs. Gross's behavior was triggered by a new, undiagnosed medical problem. Because of her dementia she could not tell anyone that she was in pain. She could only mumble and cry. Since this was not normal behavior for her, a physical exam was performed, and a bowel obstruction was discovered. The obstruction caused a great deal of pain, and it was the cause of her crying. Thus, it was not the bathing technique that was the problem but an expression of an unmet physical need.*

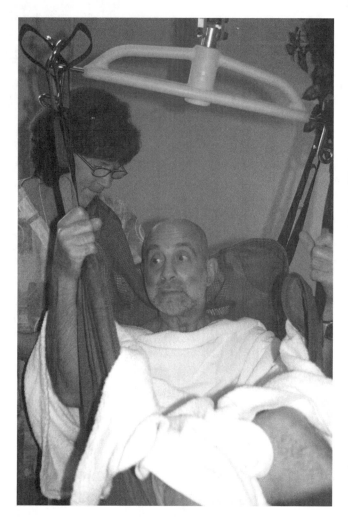

FIGURE 4.2 Fearful experience of the lift.

Emotional needs include:

- *Feeling safe and secure:* Many factors can cause the person being bathed to be afraid. Areas to explore include fear of the lift or of falling during transfer, fear of a new caregiver or of an unfamiliar environment, or fear of unexplained noises in the bathing room. Watch for signals of fear such as a fearful facial expression (wide-open eyes, open or tensed mouth, eyebrows in a straight line), an effort to get away from the caregiver or bathroom, or a refusal to enter the bathroom or shower area. Figure 4.2 illustrates this.
- *Freedom from mood or sleep problems:* Depression can be difficult to diagnose in persons with dementia. However, untreated depression can cause emotional pain. Look for the following signs of depression: sleep disturbance, poor appetite, restlessness, irritability, complaints of tiredness, feel-

ings of worthlessness or guilt, and lack of interest in other things or people. If the person is depressed, is he on a large enough dose of antidepressant to decrease symptoms? Have the underlying causes of depression been explored?
- *Respect for beliefs about modesty:* Many elderly persons have never been comfortable being naked. Watch for efforts to keep covered or exclamations of concern when private areas are uncovered or touched.
- *Feeling a sense of control:* All persons need to feel they have control over what happens to them. When a person loses even the ability to control when and how he will be touched, undressed, or washed, it is devastating. This is often expressed in demands, threats, or refusal to cooperate.

TABLE 4.2   Possible Characteristics of Persons With Mild, Moderate, and Severe Dementia

	Mild	Moderate	Severe
Orientation	Some disorientation to time	Oriented to name only	Disoriented in all spheres
Memory	Unable to recall some major, old information and learn new information	Can recognize familiar people Largely unaware of recent events Sketchy knowledge of past life Generally unaware of surroundings/seasons	No recognizable memory
ADLs (Activities of Daily Living)	No assistance needed with toileting and eating, some assistance needed with choosing proper clothing	Needs some assistance with all ADLs Becomes incontinent	Totally dependent
Behavior/Personality	Some changes: apathetic, some suspiciousness	Repetitive, obsessive behaviors, irritability, fidgety, psychosis, sleep disturbances	Extreme irritability
Problem Solving/Judgment	Impaired planning and decision making	Severely impaired: unable to understand limitations or consequences of actions	No discernible ability, unable to problem solve
Language	Word-finding problems	Language usually becomes "word salad" as disease progresses	All verbal abilities lost
Mobility	Unimpaired	Ambulatory until end of this stage; may be restless	Unable to walk, sit, or (eventually) to hold up head
Attention	Slightly reduced	Easily distracted and some trouble starting or stopping task	Severely impaired
Perception	Mild problems in new areas	Unable to recognize common objects and environmental cues	Severely impaired

Dementia-related problems: People with Alzheimer's disease and related problems often develop symptoms to which the caregiver must adjust. Often, as the disease progresses, a person is unable to communicate needs or to understand what is happening. Changes in the person's mental and functional abilities may be subtle and may occur over time. How this occurs varies from person to person. However, organizing these changes into the three stages of Alzheimer's disease can sometimes be helpful in understanding the disease. The changes are summarized in Table 4.2.

Often different kinds of behavioral symptoms arise at different stages of dementia. For example, a person with mild dementia is more likely to verbally refuse a bath by saying: "I've already had a bath." Persons with moderate dementia may say "Stop!" or firmly hold the doorjamb and refuse to enter the bathroom. Persons with severe cognitive limitations may moan or cry when they enter the bathroom. Examples of dementia-related behaviors and possible strategies for addressing them are in Table 4.3.

When assessing a person's strengths and dementia-related problems, get answers to the following questions:

- How does the person communicate? Is she able to tell you what is wrong? Can she understand simple words or do you need to use gestures and physical guidance to help the person understand?
- What problems does the person have with impulse control, judgment, and understanding events or interactions?
- How is the person's hearing and vision? Is there an impairment that may contribute to a lack of understanding? Can noise and distractions be reduced to enhance sensory input and understanding?
- Can the person perform routine tasks without assistance? How much help is needed? (See chapter 6, Person-Directed Care: Sustaining Interactions Through Offering the Needed Level of Assistance, for a detailed discussion of the assessment of the appropriate level of assistance.)

TABLE 4.3   Dementia-Related Behaviors

Cognitive Skill	Example	Action
Memory	Says: "I already had a bath" Failure to recognize caregiver Person stops during a bathing step	Avoid arguing or reasoning Use the same caregiver every day Gently remind person of next step
Language Communication	Unable to understand what others say Unable to put thoughts into words	Keep it simple Use gestures or modeling Keep your body language open and friendly Use visual props and cues to augment words Match your words and body language Make frequent eye contact if culturally appropriate Anticipate the person's needs Give the person your undivided attention
Perception Problems	Failure to recognize objects such as washcloth or soap Misinterprets environmental cues and has difficulty adjusting to new places Inability to judge depth such as that of the tub, afraid to step over the side	Hand the person the object and use physical guidance to show how to use it Explain every step Use frequent reassurance Keep environment stable If the person seems to be afraid of falling, give extra support and reassurance
Motor Functioning	Inability to perform spontaneous movements Inability to stop or start a task	Explain every step, use physical guidance Use physical guidance to help the person get started
Judgment	Accuses caregivers of interfering and refuses to cooperate with requests Responds to requests with fear and anxiety	Try to anticipate problem areas Avoid confrontation Stop at the first sign of negative emotion and try to figure out what is going on Explain what you are doing at all times and avoid surprises Limit choices
Attention	Short attention span and easily distracted	Repeat verbal prompts Use touch to get the person's attention Give simple one-step instructions Never leave the person unattended in the bath or shower Make eye contact Eliminate distractions
Body Orientation	Unable to identify body parts Unable to understand the difference between right and left	Use gestures (pointing and motioning) Use physical guidance when gesturing Give simple verbal prompts Avoid instructions such as "raise your right arm" Use verbal prompts along with touch

Additional content contributed by C. G. Rapp, V. Shue, and C. Beck.

Adapting to Personal Factors

When Mrs. Peters was invited to bathe by Paula, her caregiver, she would shake her fist and threaten Paula. She would shout that she had already had her bath and that she wanted to be left alone. Mrs. Peters was in the early stages of dementia. Her language skills were good, and she could bathe herself, but her memory and judgment were poor. Her bath time was usually around 10 a.m. after she had already dressed for the day and had her breakfast. She did not remember that she had not had a bath, and she did not realize that she was dirty. Trying to convince her only made matters worse, and she would become more insistent that she had already taken a bath.

Discussion: Several personal factors are triggering Mrs. Peters's aggressive response. These include dementia-related factors and a need to feel a sense of control. To adapt to both, Paula avoided arguing with her. She approached Mrs. Peters before she had dressed and chatted with her about her farm duties, using information she knew about her personal history. Once she had established a rapport with Mrs. Peters, Paula asked her if she would like to get ready for her day. Mrs. Peters responded yes, went willingly to the shower room, and washed herself. A battle was avoided because Paula found a way to give Mrs. Peters a sense of control and to use her remaining skills. She never mentioned the word bath but used Mrs. Peters's language of "getting ready for the day." Mrs. Peters viewed Paula's invitation to the bath as questioning her judgment. Mrs. Peters was offended by the suggestion that she was dirty and hadn't cleaned herself, so she felt she had to defend herself. Paula also took the time to create a friendly, validating relationship by talking with Mrs. Peters about the things she used to do on her farm.

Consider Relationship/Interpersonal Factors

Your behavior can often unknowingly trigger distress. When you become aware of the effect of your behavior and change your approach, behavioral symptoms often decrease. Pay particular attention to your own nonverbal messages. They are conveyed through tone of voice, facial expressions, and gestures, which often communicate more than words. Be sure that your nonverbal messages match your words and that they convey caring. Answer the following questions to determine what interpersonal factors might be contributing to the person's distress.

- Do you repeatedly respond to complaints of pain or cold, apologize, and take some action? (Persons with dementia may not process or remember your responses and may need frequent repetitions.)
- Are there too many people in the bathroom? Could this be overwhelming?
- Are you talking with someone else in the room or are you focused on the person being bathed? Are you using a friendly, calm approach with good eye contact, if culturally appropriate?
- Do you explain each step in simple language and match your communication to the person's abilities?
- Do you smile often?
- Are you moving too fast for this person?
- Are you trying to do too much at one time?
- Do you acknowledge and respect the person's need for privacy?
- Do you consider gender preferences?

Focusing on the Relationship

Mrs. Johns resisted bathing. Her caregiver, Rose, learned from Mrs. Johns's family that she had loved to shop. Rose brought in a catalogue for Mrs. Johns to look at while she was being washed with a no-rinse soap and water. She would ask Mrs. Johns what she liked best on each page and would create a fun experience for both of them. Whenever Mrs. Johns complained, Rose would apologize and take corrective action.

Discussion: Rose has a positive, interpersonal approach. She focuses on the person she is bathing and makes the bath a pleasurable experience. She makes an effort to get to know the person. She uses personal information about Mrs. Johns to help distract her from an unpleasant task. Rather than focusing on the washing task, Rose pays close attention to Mrs. Johns's needs. She is quick to apologize and change her approach, if possible. Rose's residents feel connected to her and well cared for.

Assess for Stressful Factors in the Physical Environment

Areas to explore in the physical environment include:

- *Lighting:* Is there enough lighting for an older person's eyes? Is it nonglare? Does the person squint when entering the bathroom?
- *Temperature:* Is the room warm enough? Is the person shivering or trying to stay covered? Is the person complaining about being cold? Is there a heat lamp in the bathing room?
- *Seating and mobility devices:* Is the equipment comfortable and fitted to the person? Does the person cry out or wince when placed on the shower chair? Does the person squirm in the shower chair, lean to the side, or attempt to get up? Does the person's bottom sink into the hole in the shower chair? Are the person's legs supported? Is the person frightened when placed on a lift?
- *Space:* Is the area cluttered, making it frightening or difficult to maneuver?
- *Noise level:* Can you hear unpleasant or unusual noises when you're in the bathroom? Is the person disturbed by these noises? Does running water make conversation difficult? Is the person having difficulty hearing you? Do you have pleasant, person-specific music playing?
- *Homelike atmosphere:* Is the bathroom institutional looking? Does the person fail to recognize that it is a bathroom? Is there adequate privacy?
- *Odors:* Are there unpleasant odors in the room? Are the room sprays being used pleasant or unpleasant? Does the person seem to be reacting to them?

Assessing Physical Factors

Mrs. Smith is a thin, frail 93-year-old with a history of hip fracture, arthritis, and peripheral neuropathy. When the typical plastic shower chair with the large hole and no foot support is used, her bottom sinks in the chair, putting pressure on her fractured hip and arthritic joints. Her legs hang as deadweight, and her feet turn blue as she complains bitterly of pain in her bottom, hip, and legs.

Discussion: Mrs. Smith is a good example of factors in the physical environment causing her discomfort. The room is cold and the equipment does not fit her body, triggering her complaints. She needs a more comfortable seating device, a footstool, and extra covering to keep her warm. When a child's padded potty-seat insert is placed in the shower chair, her feet are supported on a small stool, and she is well-covered, her complaints decrease dramatically.

Assess the Organizational Environment

Rigid administrative policies and practices can hamper your ability to provide individualized care. Assess the following areas for possible discomfort triggers:

- *Philosophy:* Does the philosophy of care allow flexibility in determining when, how, and who will be bathed? When persons are distressed, are you criticized if you postpone some tasks and clean only essential areas?
- *Policies and procedures:* Is there a policy that dictates the frequency and types of baths? Can you substitute a bed bath for a shower?
- *Supervision and staffing patterns:* How many different caregivers might bathe a person each month? Do staffing patterns support individualized care? Are caregivers rotated among groups so that they do not care for the same person every day? Are there consistent assignments so direct caregivers get to know the people they care for?
- *Structure of the day:* Are all baths expected to be done in the morning? Are staff on all shifts encouraged to adjust when baths are given to meet the habits and preferences of individuals?
- *Staff support and education:* Are nursing assistants taught a rigid procedure for showering, and does their training reinforce flexibility and individualization? What strategies are taught for coping with agitation and aggression? Is distress during bathing considered normal for persons with dementia or is it seen as a need for further assessment and intervention?
- *Equipment and supplies:* Is there a wide variety of bathing supplies available to meet individual needs? Is there a limit to the supplies that can be used for one bath?

Rigid Rules

Mrs. Jones is a 60-year-old woman with mild dementia. She refuses to shower and she states that she "doesn't like a shower." She cannot elaborate on her reasons, but she is adamant in her refusal. The nursing home where she resides requires two showers a week. She must be forced to shower, resulting in self-protective behaviors such as hitting and kicking. Sometimes it takes four staff members to shower her. This is very upsetting to all involved.

Discussion: Mrs. Jones illustrates the problems caused by rigid policies. When the two showers a week rule is discontinued, alternative bathing methods can be tried. An in-bed towel bath was tried, and Mrs. Jones responded favorably. She called it her "steam bath," and she smiled and was very cooperative. She was clean and happy. Meeting the individual needs of persons with dementia requires flexibility.

SUMMARY

A behavior such as yelling can have many causes and will respond to different solutions depending upon whether the cause is personal, interpersonal, environmental, or a combination of factors. If you think the person's distress is caused by cold, you can assess for personal factors such as decreased body fat, a history of sensitivity to cold, or circulatory problems. Next, assess the environment. Check the room temperature. Also, look at how you respond to the person's behavior. Do you try to keep him covered? Do you acknowledge complaints of cold?

Understanding causes or triggers for behavioral symptoms that occur during bathing is the first step in stopping the bathing battle. This helps you tailor your approach to the individual needs of the person you are bathing and make it person-directed. Gather as much information as you can about the person. Then select one behavior that suggests that the person is uncomfortable. Look for the trigger(s) for this behavior by assessing the physical, emotional, and dementia-related needs of the person, the quality of the interaction during the bath, and the characteristics of the physical and organizational environments. The information you gather will help you select the solutions to improve the bathing experience.

APPENDIX
PERSONAL HISTORY

The forms on the following pages can help you understand behavior and help you develop bathing routines that are tailored to the unique needs of each individual. They include:

- **Personal Information Data Sheet:** Use this form for helpful information about the person's past and current life (see Figure 4.3).
- **Bathing Preferences and Practices Form:** This can be sent to the family to learn about prior bathing habits (see Figure 4.4).

Personal Information Data Sheet

Name _____

Nickname _____

Occupation _____

Past Accomplishments _____

Education _____

Current Interests/Activities _____

Hobbies, Topics of Interest _____

Family: Spouse   Yes ☐ No ☐   Name _____

         Children   Yes ☐ No ☐   Name(s)_____

Other Regular Visitors _____

Favorite Foods _____

Favorite Music _____

Level of Dementia

         Able to Understand Words?   Yes ☐   No ☐

         Able to Remember   _____ Family _____ Caregiver _____ Events

         Difficulty With Judgment   Yes ☐   No ☐

         Able to Help With Bath   Yes ☐   No ☐

Personality _____

Current Medical Problems _____

Pain Site, If Any

_____ Back   _____ Hips   _____ Feet   _____ Head

Other (Where?) _____

Spiritual Beliefs/Religion _____

Cultural Beliefs/Prejudices _____

Language _____

Summary From Bathing Preferences Form _____

_____

FIGURE 4.3   Personal information data sheet.

In order to better care for _____,
we would like to learn about his/her bathing history and
preferences. We would appreciate you providing as much
information as possible.

Your name: _____

Relationship to resident: _____

The following questions are about _____'s
bathing habits. Please describe his/her habits both before the
disease and after by checking one box in the "before illness"
column and one in the "after illness" column.

1. How many times each week did he/she bathe?

		Before Illness	After Illness
less than once/week		☐	☐
1-2 times/wk		☐	☐
3-4 times/wk		☐	☐
more than 4 times/wk		☐	☐

2. What time of day did he/she bathe? (Check all that apply)

		Before Illness	After Illness
before 7 a.m.		☐	☐
morning		☐	☐
afternoon		☐	☐
evening		☐	☐
just before bed		☐	☐

3. How long was his/her bath?

		Before Illness	After Illness
less than 10 minutes		☐	☐
15-30 minutes		☐	☐
30-60 minutes		☐	☐
more than 1 hour		☐	☐

4. Where did he/she bathe?

		Before Illness	After Illness
bathtub		☐	☐
shower		☐	☐
sponge bath		☐	☐

5. Which bathing items were used? (check all that apply)

☐ washcloth
☐ sponge
☐ brush
☐ special soap (what kind?): _____
☐ other (describe): _____

6. Describe the way he/she rinsed the soap:

☐ with water from the shower nozzle
☐ with remaining bath-water in tub
☐ using a bathside commode/basin
☐ other (describe): _____

7. Did he/she use talcum powder after bathing?

_____ No   _____ Yes (what kind): _____

8. Did he/she use moisturizing lotion?

_____ No   _____ Yes (what kind): _____

9. Describe his/her feeling about bathing in general?

		Before Illness	After Illness
strongly dislikes		☐	☐
mildly dislikes		☐	☐
neutral		☐	☐
likes		☐	☐
strongly likes		☐	☐

10. How was taking a bath started (after illness began)?

☐ he/she started it by himself/herself
☐ you suggested it once
☐ you suggested it several times
☐ only by physically bringing him/her to the bathing area

FIGURE 4.4 Bathing preferences and practices form.

The following questions are about _____'s ability to bathe himself/herself immediately before admission. Please describe the help you or another caregiver provided, if any.

1. Describe his/her ability to get undressed for the bath:

   ☐ He/she needs no help
   ☐ Undressed self with encouragement
   ☐ You helped with less than half of the undressing
   ☐ You did it all

2. Did you prepare the bath for him/her (turn on water to fill a basin)?

   _____ No   _____ Yes

3. Describe his/her ability to get in the bath or shower:

   ☐ He/she needs no help
   ☐ He/she got in with encouragement
   ☐ You helped with less than half
   ☐ You helped with more than half
   ☐ You put him/her in

4. Describe his/her ability to wash herself:

   ☐ He/she needs no help
   ☐ Undressed self with encouragement
   ☐ You helped with less than half the washing
   ☐ You helped with more than half the washing
   ☐ You did it all

5. Describe how he/she dried herself:

   ☐ He/she needs no help
   ☐ He/she dried self with encouragement
   ☐ You helped with less than half the drying
   ☐ You helped with more than half the drying
   ☐ You did it all

6. Describe his/her ability to get dressed after the bath:

   ☐ He/she needs no help
   ☐ He/she dressed self with encouragement
   ☐ You helped with less than half the dressing
   ☐ You helped with more than half the dressing
   ☐ You did it all

Your answers to the following will help us find ways to make bathing a safer, easier, and more enjoyable activity for all residents and staff. Please give as much information as you can.

1. Please tell us about any problems you faced while bathing (undressing, getting in and out of the tub, washing, drying, or dressing).

2. Can you give us any "special tips" that you found helpful in bathing? Please describe all the things you did or said that helped make the bathing process easier and more pleasurable either for you or him/her.

Thank you very much for taking time to answer these questions

Developed by S. Dwyer, A. L. Barrick, and P. D. Sloan (University of North Carolina at Chapel Hill) as part of the research grant, Reducing Disruptive Behaviors in Dementia During Bathing (R01 AG11506), funded by the National Institute on Aging. This form may be reproduced for clinical, research, or teaching purposes.

FIGURE 4.4 (*continued*)

CHAPTER 5

Selecting Person-Directed Solutions That Work[1]

Ann Louise Barrick, Joanne Rader, Madeline Mitchell

To increase comfort during the bath you need to develop a realistic, person-directed care plan that addresses the personal needs, preferences, and abilities identified in your assessment. In addition, you may need to modify the environment. All this requires thought and planning. After your assessment, the next two steps in the process are selecting solutions to try and testing these solutions. Refer to the Intervention Planning Table (see Appendix A) as a tool to help you develop and implement your plan.

Set Realistic Expectations

For most persons with dementia, the goal of making bathing pleasurable or at least tolerable is realistic. For others with dementia, bathing is extremely upsetting, and only small improvements in comfort are possible. For these individuals the best you can do is provide some distraction and a slight decrease in discomfort. For example, we worked with one woman who yelled and tried to hit the caregiver every time she was touched. We tried different kinds of baths and interventions. Only distraction and a very gentle, slow, supportive approach, stopping every time she started to yell or strike at us, seemed to help. We could distract her by having her hold and comfort a doll and by using a second nursing assistant to talk with her. With these efforts we were able to clean her and slightly decrease discomfort expressed by yelling and hitting.

Establish the Goals for the Bath

In addition to the general goal of wanting the bath to be more pleasurable, you need to identify and select one specific behavior to address. Does the person yell? Hit? Try to bite? How often does this happen? Identify behavioral changes that will let you know when the person is less distressed. You can define your goal in terms of a reduction in these behavioral symptoms and/or an increase in signs of pleasure. Will it be a decrease in complaints of being cold from 7–10 per bath to less than 3 per bath? Will it be a decrease in the percentage of time the person makes a wailing noise during bathing? Will the best measure be an increase in the number of times the person smiles during the shower or the fact that he smiles at all? Table 5.1 gives examples of various goals and how to measure them.

For example, we worked with a gentleman who always cried out whenever we tried to wash him. He had been a minister and liked to sing. Any time he began to yell, his caregiver stopped what she was doing, quieted her tone, used gentle touch, and asked him if he would sing a hymn for her. The singing calmed his anxieties, distracted him, and created a way for him to be of service to others. The more he sang, the less he yelled! This was a good measure of success.

If a person becomes distressed when being bathed you have to ask yourself what really needs to be cleaned now. What areas are dirty? What tasks can be done another time? For example, hair washing can be very distressing. If the person's hair does not look greasy, it is best to postpone that task until another day. In another example, Mrs. Brown was upset just at the mention of the word "bath." The usual routine was to shower, wash her hair, cut her toenails and fingernails, and brush her teeth as part of the same bathing experience. She became increasingly upset during the course of the "bath." She began by saying no, then she started to cry and escalated to trying to hit her caregiver. When her hair, nails, and

TABLE 5.1 Setting Measurable Goals

Behaviors	Goal	How Measured
Distressed Behaviors		
Pinching	Reduce by 50%	Decrease pinching from 6 times per bath to 3 by (date)
Crying out	Reduce by 75%	Decrease episodes from 20 to 5 per bath
Screams when bottom washed	No screaming	Record if screaming did or did not occur during task
Positive Behaviors		
Engaging in conversation	Respond to questions	Will respond to at least 2 questions per bath
Sings with caregiver	Person will sing when caregiver initiates, showing an increase in comfort	Person will sing once per bath from current once per 4 baths
Thanks caregiver	Person will be comfortable during bathing	Person expresses appreciation for help. Smiles, laughs, or hugs caregiver during 3 consecutive baths

teeth were done at a different time, there was a noticeable improvement in her comfort level as shown by a reduction in complaints and elimination of the hitting behavior. The routine of getting it all done at once was altered to avoid the battle.

Determine the Level of Independence

Involving the person in the bath and having her wash those parts that she can may help make the bath more pleasurable. Ask yourself these questions: Can this person do any part of the bath herself? What level of assistance is needed to maximize independence and minimize unnecessary disability? How much does the person *want* to be independent?

However, encouraging independence in someone unable to perform a task may increase agitation. Understanding the level of dementia and specific deficits will help you select strategies that fit the person's abilities. During the course of our study, as the nursing assistant developed a relationship with the person, we were often surprised by the emergence of previously hidden abilities to do self-care such as washing one's own face, chest, and "private parts," even among severely impaired persons. Different techniques seem to work better depending on the person's level of dementia. For example, the milder the dementia is, the more useful are the techniques of talking with the person, asking her to help, or giving choices. See chapter 6, Person-Directed Care: Sustaining Interactions Through Offering the Needed Level of Assistance, for a detailed discussion of methods for choosing the best level of assistance.

Persons in the later stages of dementia tend to respond well to physical guidance and distractions such as something to hold, look at, or eat or drink. Of course, it is essential when working with persons with dementia to assess whether they are likely to try to place objects in their mouths that could cause choking. When you are providing food or drink, it is critical to be aware of swallowing and dietary precautions and to make choices that are pleasing to the individual but also safe.

Determine the Level of Communication to Use

Ask yourself, what can the person understand? It is important to use the person's vocabulary. If the person uses the word "poop" to describe having a bowel movement, that is the word you should use when talking to him. Adapt your communication style to the person's level of understanding. For example, use verbal interventions with a person who can understand simple language. However, nonverbal interventions such as food or other distracting objects are helpful for a person with more advanced dementia and no verbal language. Examples of distracters are in Table 5.2.

Select Solutions that Meet Specific Needs

Your job is to fit the solution to the person. Choose those strategies that address the possible causes of behavioral symptoms. Because behaviors are so complicated and can have different triggers you often have to try many different things to discover what makes the person the

TABLE 5.2 Sample Distracters

Food	Conversation	Objects to Hold	Others
Cookies	About family	A towel	Music
Gum	About food	A washcloth	A balloon to observe
Crackers	About pets	A stuffed animal	A plant to observe
Lollipops	About the farm	Your hand	A mobile
Bananas	About past work	A small figurine	
Peppermints	How attractive they are	A sponge	
Chocolate	Ask questions	A ball	
Coffee	Ask opinions	A mirror	
Tea	Give praise	A doll	
Cake			

most comfortable. For example, if the person appears to be cold (e.g., yells, grabs clothing as you try to remove it) you can use both environmental and interpersonal solutions. Try warming the room before bringing the person to the bathing room. When the person complains of being cold, cover him, apologize, and reassure him that you will make every effort to keep him warm. At other times you may want to try one solution at a time. For example, if the person appears to be afraid of falling you may begin by reassuring him often in a calm, soothing voice. Next you can try using a different type of transfer (see chapter 9, Transfer Techniques). If this does not decrease his distress, you may want to try a bed bath instead of a shower and eliminate the trigger for his fear.

In another example, you may think that pain is the cause of a person's yelling. You know the person's feet are very sensitive, and she seems to yell most when you are washing them. You may want to wash her feet last so you do not upset him. Or you can try soaking her feet first to loosen dirt and gently use the edge of a baby washcloth to wash between the toes. Apologize at any sign of pain.

Success usually requires great creativity and persistence. It may take 3–4 weeks to find the right combination of solutions. There is no "cookbook" for bathing. Each solution must be carefully selected. Music can provide distraction and relaxation. But you have to know the person's preferences and use very specific types of music with each person—country western for some, classical for others. Similarly, food and objects you choose for the person to hold or look at need to be selected based on your knowledge of the person and trial and error. The following case study illustrates this process.

Case Study

Mrs. Swanson did not enjoy her routine showers. She often said she did not want to go and almost constantly cried and complained of being cold and being in pain. She asked staff to hurry up. Sometimes she mixed words up, saying, for example, that the water was too hot when she really meant too cold.

Before helping her, we reviewed what we knew or what we could locate in the chart about her. She was 93 years old and very proud of having been a preacher's wife. She also made women's hats and liked fashion. She had been very active in the church, and her beliefs remained a source of support for her. Mrs. Swanson had done a lot of handwork, such as embroidery, and she enjoyed cooking and baking. She had entered the nursing home 2 years before after fracturing her hip. Her diagnoses included Alzheimer's disease, arthritis, peripheral neuropathy (from diabetes), and limited vision and hearing. She was incontinent of both urine and stool.

Her history included many possible sources of pain—arthritis, her previous hip fracture, peripheral neuropathy, and possibly some undiagnosed illness. We noted that Mrs. Swanson had an order for acetaminophen four times a day as necessary for pain, but that she rarely received it.

As we began to work with her, we tried to view the bath from her perspective. We noticed that she was transferred using a two-person underarm assist. We also noted that during this process her face was anxious, and she complained of pain. In the bathroom, we noticed that the bathing chair was a standard one, made of plastic pipe with a hard seat, and that the room temperature was cool. After this initial assessment, we felt her major sources of distress came from her needs for comfort, warmth, and security.

Based on this assessment, we focused on trying to reduce pain and increase warmth. We asked that the acetaminophen be given routinely and made sure that she got a dose early in the morning so that it would be working by the time we assisted her in the shower. We cushioned the shower chair with a padded seat and warmed the shower room by turning on the heat lamp before bringing her in. We kept her covered with towels while showering, lifting the towels to wash small areas, and rinsed her body with a hand-held nozzle. In addition, we played church music to distract and relax her, though it was difficult to know how much she understood because of her hearing loss and the fact that the music echoed in the bathroom.

Her complaints decreased, but the shower was not yet a pleasant experience for her. So we renewed our efforts and tried some other things. We asked that she be given additional pain medication (a narcotic) prior to the shower. But her pain complaints, mostly related to being moved, did not change; and the medication only made her drowsy. Looking again at the physical environment, we decided we would no longer use the hand-held shower to rinse her, since the water spray seemed to trigger and increase her discomfort and her leg pain. So we started washing her with baby washcloths, using a no-rinse soap solution in a basin, and we kept her covered and warm the entire time, lifting the towels to wash.

At the same time, the nursing assistant experimented with techniques of distraction when Mrs. Swanson appeared anxious. They sang hymns together; "The Old Rugged Cross" was a favorite. She gave Mrs. Swanson small plastic figurines to hold and to comment on or talked about her son or her work in the church. This worked well when used just before a difficult procedure, such as washing her buttocks and genital area. Before the nursing assistant touched an area that might be painful, she told Mrs. Swanson she was going to touch her and that she would be careful. If Mrs. Swanson complained of pain or being cold, the nursing assistant would apologize and take some action to address her need, such as covering an area or readjusting her in the shower chair. We also soaked her feet in a basin of water while we washed her in the shower, and she found this soothing.

To help make transfers less painful, we consulted with a physical therapist who suggested trying a sliding board transfer, going slow and explaining the moves step by step. This decreased Mrs. Swanson's complaints slightly. Our "best guess" was that fear and anxiety were also playing a role, so we added new solutions. We asked her to count with us before we started the transfer; this yielded fewer complaints of pain and fear.

A surprisingly effective intervention during the shower was to give her a mirror to hold. The nursing assistant thought of this idea, remembering that Mrs. Swanson always looked in the hall mirror when she was transported in the wheelchair down the hall. As Mrs. Swanson held the mirror, the nursing assistant would comment about how nice she was going to look after the bath.

Because Mrs. Swanson disliked having her hair washed, we did this last, taking care to keep her warm and well-covered. We wet her head with washcloths, using minimal shampoo. We carefully poured from a small graduate pitcher, avoiding her face and ears. This, along with talking to her about topics of interest, made the hair washing more pleasant for her. At the same time, we shared simple jokes with her, and sometimes we could get her to laugh.

This was a trial-and-error process. The result was a person-directed bathing care plan that worked for Mrs. Swanson (Table 5.3). Measurable improvements included the following behaviors:

- She agreed to the shower.
- She no longer cried in the shower.
- Her complaints of pain decreased from 10 per bath to less than 5 per bath.
- Her complaints of being cold decreased from 15 per bath to less than 3.
- She showed interest in objects she was holding.
- She would thank the nursing assistant for her help.

Reaching these goals required getting to know her, viewing the shower through her eyes, modifying the environment, and meeting her needs for comfort and security. This required ongoing thinking and planning, but the final result took no additional time for the nursing assistant and was much more pleasant for Mrs. Swanson.

Tables 5.4 to 5.16 list specific behaviors that might occur during bathing and suggest possible reasons and solutions, looking holistically at factors that may be personal, relational, part of the physical or organizational environment. These tables can be useful in identifying a wide variety of solutions to try when making your approach person-directed. Once you have chosen a behavior, consult the appropriate table. Find the possible cause you have determined for the behavior, then select a solution to try.

TABLE 5.3   Person-Directed Shower Care Plan for Mrs. Swanson

Needs Identified:

For comfort—has pain particularly in her legs and feet
To be warm
To feel safe

Behavioral Symptoms:

Crying, complaints of being cold, in pain
Refusing shower

Goals:

Increase comfort related to transfers and foot and leg pain
Decrease fear and anxiety and increase pleasure
Keep her warm

Suggested Approaches:

To increase comfort and warmth:

- Give routine Tylenol 1 hour before shower
- Give shower before breakfast
- Assess her level of discomfort before you begin
- Turn on heat lamp in shower room to warm it
- Pad shower chair with child potty seat insert
- Move her carefully and slowly
- Tell her before you touch her, especially her feet; touch legs gently and move legs up and down gently before beginning transfer
- Use sliding board transfer
- Go slowly and ask her to count with you before transfer
- Use touch and soothing voice to reassure her you care and that you understand that she hurts
- Position her carefully in shower chair
- Keep her well-covered throughout shower, lifting towel to wash areas; use basin with washcloths and no-rinse soap solution instead of water spray
- Sincerely apologize if she complains of pain, being cold
- Try singing hymns with her
- Distract her with objects such as a hand mirror, cute figurines

To decrease fear and anxiety:

- Distract her with conversation on favorite topics—her son, the church
- Speak clearly and distinctly, making eye contact as much as possible so she can read lips
- Explain any misunderstanding she has related to being hard of hearing (e.g., She hears "watch" instead of "wash")
- Respond quickly to her complaints of being cold by adding blankets, etc.
- Wash hair last—be sure she is warm and well-covered with bath blanket before beginning; wet head with washcloths; use a small amount of baby shampoo; rinse using a small amount of water from small pitcher or graduate, deflecting water from face and ears

TABLE 5.4 Tips for When the Person Doesn't Want to Come to the Bathing Area

Possible Reason	Action	Explanation
Personal		
Doesn't want to bathe right now	Try later	Person may not be feeling up to it now
Fear	Approach person alone	A crowd of people may seem threatening
Control	Offer a reward. Try a favorite activity or food	A treat makes bathing seem less unpleasant and can provide motivation to bathe
	Invite the person for a walk without mentioning "bath"	Distracts person and avoids struggle
	Ask if the person would prefer a tub, shower, or bed bath	Give person a choice and a feeling of control
Interpersonal/Relationship		
Doesn't recognize you	Try another caregiver, or invite a family member to help	Person may prefer a different caregiver or someone with whom she has a closer relationship
Doesn't trust you	Walk or talk with the person for a few minutes before inviting the person to bathe	Builds trust prior to asking the person to do something
Physical		
Unfamiliar environment	Assess if someone or something in the bathing area is contributing to the refusal	Aspects of the room, such as lighting, temperature, or another resident may provoke refusal
	Bathe in another location, such as in own room	Avoids transferring person to an unfamiliar or scary place. Person may be more comfortable in her own room
Uncomfortable equipment	Try different transportation method, such as a wheelchair	Person may want or need some assistance

TABLE 5.5   Tips for When the Person Doesn't Want to Bathe

Possible Reason	Action	Explanation
Personal		
Pain	Invite the person to the bath after pain meds have had a chance to alleviate person's discomfort	Relief of pain associated with transfer, transport, and bath-related tasks may change how the person feels about the possibility of a bath
	Use a different method of transfer	
	Use a bed bath	Bed baths avoid painful transfers
Person has difficulty with transitions—leaving one location or activity for another	Take advantage of natural transition times. Invite the person into the bathing area when the person walks by it and/or is already up and about	Is less disruptive to person
Person needs incentives for bathing	Offer a reward: Try a favorite activity or food	A treat makes bathing seem less unpleasant and can be motivating
Person may not be feeling up to it now	Try later	The initial reaction may be a passing sentiment. Acknowledging the person's feelings may affect how the person responds. Gives him some control
Person has difficulty with mobility	Use a wheelchair or other device to help the person get to the shower	Walking to the bath may be very tiring/painful for some people
Interpersonal/Relationship		
Person may not understand that he/she needs a bath	Create a reason: Say it is time to freshen up for an activity, work, or visitors; tell the person that his clothes look uncomfortable or need to be changed	Person may want to know why it is time to bathe
	Walk or talk with the person for a few minutes before inviting to bathe	Builds trust prior to asking person to do something
Person has caregiver preferences	Delay until preferred caregiver is available.	Person may prefer a different caregiver or someone with whom he/she has a closer relationship
	Try another caregiver, or invite a family member to help. If a preference cannot be honored, talk to the person about that. Are there gender issues?	Acknowledgment of preferences can positively affect a person's response to a less desirable situation
Person needs a quiet approach	Approach the person alone	Even two people may seem threatening to some persons

(continued)

TABLE 5.5 (*Continued*)

Possible Reason	Action	Explanation
Physical Environment		
Room temperature or water temperature	Check room temperature before bringing person for bathing; check water temperature frequently	Older persons may be especially sensitive to temperature variations
Noise	Reduce amount of noise or conversation with anyone other than the person being bathed	Multiple sensory events can be disturbing to a cognitively impaired person
Privacy	Keep person covered as much as possible. Bathe only one person at a time	Feels safer and more respectful of privacy needs
Device used to transport person is uncomfortable	Try a different transportation method. Add cushions or other padding for comfort or positioning	Provides increased comfort and support for the person, resulting in less resistance
Uncomfortable shower chair	Use an appropriately sized chair, and/or use water-resistant cushions; pad chair	Small individuals may not get adequate support in a large shower chair. Large persons may feel cramped. Pads provide cushioning and additional support
Organizational Environment		
Time of day	Determine if person prefers to be bathed at a particular time of day. Use information when setting up bath schedule	Natural body rhythms vary among individuals. Accommodating these variations may change how a person reacts to the prospect of a bath
Mode of bathing	Determine whether the person would prefer a tub, shower, or bed bath. If the person is unable to respond, talk to other staff and/or family members. Try different ways of bathing and monitor results	Accommodates person's preference. Also, gives a choice and a feeling of control

TABLE 5.6 Tips for When the Person Doesn't Want to Get Undressed

Possible Reason	Action	Explanation
Personal		
Control	Have person choose clothes to be worn after the bath	Gives a sense of control over what is happening
	Create a reason: Say "You'll look nice in clean clothes" or "your clothes are dirty"	Gives a reason to undress
	Praise helping efforts	Encourages assistance
	Accept the refusal and offer to check back later	Gives a sense of control/autonomy
	Offer choices: "Shall I undo your belt or do you want to?"	Allows some control over events
Fear	Reassure often	May feel attacked. Helps feel more secure
	Explain what you are doing in very simple words	May feel attacked. Helps understand
	Move slowly and gently, avoiding any "rushing" or fast movements	Going too quickly may frighten and confuse person
	Start by taking off shoes	Less threatening than taking upper body clothing off
Modesty	Undress from under a covering, such as a towel around the waist, before removing pants	Maintains privacy
Cold	Keep person covered as often as possible with towels or with a blanket	May keep from feeling cold
Interpersonal/Relationship		
Doesn't understand your request	Try gesturing or physical guidance	May help understand
	Use distraction	May help gain cooperation if person can focus on something else
Doesn't recognize you as a caregiver	Introduce yourself and give time to understand	May help gain cooperation
Physical		
Room temperature is cool	Heat room prior to asking person to undress	Helps keep the person comfortable
Organizational		
Different caregivers several times a week	Make permanent care assignments	Allows the caregiver to get to know the person well and build the relationship

TABLE 5.7 Tips for When the Person Refuses to Get Into Tub/Shower or Sit in Tub or on Shower Chair

Possible Reason	Action	Explanation
Personal		
Control	Have person test water temperature	Involves person in the activity, providing a sense of control over what is happening
	Praise helping efforts	Encourages assistance
	Bathe standing in shower using aqua socks or using PVC pipe walker or walking frame	Promotes safety and feeling of autonomy. Is more familiar way to shower
	Accept the refusal and offer to check back later	Provides sense of control and autonomy. Promotes relationship
Fear of falling	Reassure person that he/she won't fall ("We have you," "You'll be safe with me")	Person may be afraid of falling. Helps feel more secure
	Let person support self during transfer and seat using available handholds/bars	Person feels supported, in control during movements
	Get assistance if needed and appropriate	Additional support may be reassuring if person is afraid of falling
	Bathe the person standing in the tub and have person hold grab bars (maintain safety)	Avoids struggle. Helps feel more secure
	Call family to get history	May have negative fears/beliefs from past
Physical Environment		
Uncomfortable furnishings	Use chairlift or transfer bench, if available	Person may have difficulties with limb movement, and equipment may make person more comfortable
	Try a different type of bath	May be more comfortable
Bathroom looks unfamiliar, unfriendly	Create "friendlier-looking" bathrooms	Person may be less fearful
	Verbally orient person to the room and to the equipment	Person may be less fearful
Interpersonal/Relationship Issues		
Doesn't understand your request	Apply gentle pressure behind knee with a chair or with your hand to stimulate sitting	Physical cues may be more helpful than verbal ones for some persons
	Break down the task into simple, step-by-step movements; match communication level with ability	Entire action may be too complex for person to know what to do first
	Try a different kind of bath (e.g., in-room bath)	Reduces demands on person unable to understand what you are asking
Prefers a different caregiver	Try getting another person to do it	You may remind him of someone else

TABLE 5.8 Tips for When the Person Feels Pain on Movement

Possible Reason	Action	Explanation
Personal		
Pain	Distract with conversation or food	Helps the person relax and may add something pleasant to the experience. Makes it an event rather than an unpleasant task
	Bathing after pain meds have had a chance to alleviate discomfort	Relief of pain may allow a more pleasant experience
	When rolling over, roll the person onto the side that causes least discomfort	Reduces discomfort
Control	Have person hold bed rail and assist with turning	Gives the person a sense of control. Makes the move easier because person can assist
	Ask what will help and wait for a response if the person can talk	Can learn what person prefers. Helps feel connected to caregiver
Fear	Count with the person before moving	Helps the person prepare for move and give assistance rather than resistance. Distracts, and avoids surprises
	Reassure	Helps the person feel more secure
	Use soothing tone	Helps to relax
	Move slowly	Gives the person time to adjust. Promotes a feeling of security
Organizational Environment		
	Get physical therapy or occupational therapy consultant to determine best method of transfer	Transfers are complex and need to be individualized for the safety and comfort of both the staff and person
	Use two to transfer	Can move the person more gently and give needed support. Reduces discomfort

TABLE 5.9 Tips for When the Person's Skin Is Tender

Possible Reason	Action	Explanation
Personal		
Pain	Wash gently using a soft touch	Less friction reduces discomfort
	Use baby washcloths	They are softer than most washcloths
	Pat dry instead of rub	Avoids friction. Gentler on tender skin
	Start with the least sensitive area	Causes less distress
	Touch gently before beginning to wash	Helps the person adjust to touch
	Use warmed wipe on rectum	These are softer than most washcloths
Control	Ask for feedback: "Does this feel OK?"	Lets the person know you care
Physical Environment		
Uncomfortable furnishings	Pad shower chair. Try a different kind of bath	May be more comfortable. Shower spray may cause discomfort
	Tell what you are going to do before doing it	Gives person a warning so he/she will be prepared. Avoids surprises
Interpersonal/Relationship Issues		
Doesn't understand	Explain what you are doing	Helps person feel understood; builds trust

TABLE 5.10 Tips for When the Person Is Incontinent During Bath

Possible Reason	Action	Explanation
Personal		
Bath given at time of routine bowel movement or urination	Investigate bowel routine and schedule bath around it	Prevention
Physical movement stimulates elimination	Toilet first	Prevention
Physical Environment		
Shower chair stimulates bowel movement	Toilet first	Prevention is key
	Give a different type of bath	Prevention is the key
	Use a shower chair with a bucket	Prevention
	Put a Chux pad on floor	Helps with cleanup. Maintains safety
Running water stimulates elimination	Run bathwater before person enters the room	Prevention is the key
	Toilet first	Prevention is key here

TABLE 5.11 Tips for When the Person Doesn't Want Feet Washed

Possible Reason	Action	Explanation
Personal		
Pain	Soak feet in a basin while sitting in shower chair	Feels good and loosens dirt
	Place moist cotton balls on toes to soak prior to washing	Helps soften dirt for easier and less painful cleaning
	Use gloved fingers instead of a washcloth to wash feet	Can feel more like a massage. Easier to get to hard-to-reach places
	Place feet on a dry towel and cover with another small towel and pat dry	Less friction and joint pain
	Wash and dry between the toes with something thin and soft (e.g., baby washcloth, cotton swab)	Allows for more gentle action in hard-to-reach places
Control	Ask for feedback. Have person wash own feet if possible	Communicates respect; reinforces independence
	Apologize at any sign of pain	Communicates respect
Physical Environment		
Uncomfortable furnishings	Support feet and legs with a stool covered with a towel	Helps with circulation and to feel more secure

TABLE 5.12   Tips for When the Person Doesn't Want Teeth Brushed

Reason	Action	Explanation
Personal		
Pain	Use a child's toothbrush	Smaller and softer and avoids pain
	Use child's toothpaste	Tastes sweet
Fear	Warn person of upcoming sensations and explain what you are doing	Avoids surprises and gives person time to prepare
	Do one step at a time	Decreases confusion as entire action may be too complex
	Distract with conversation about family, hobbies, food	Helps to distract person and may add some pleasure to the experience
	Sing songs the person likes	Distracts person and helps him relax
	Remain calm	Reassures person
	Reassure frequently	Promotes feeling of safety
Interpersonal/Relationship		
Trust	Apologize at any sign of pain	Validates the person and helps person feel understood

TABLE 5.13 Tips for When the Person Grabs and Holds Onto Objects

Possible Reason	Action	Explanation
Personal/Interpersonal		
Pain	Support during transfers	Grabbing may reflect pain
	Try a different type bath	Avoids transfers or lifting that may cause pain
Does not understand	Give person something to hold such as a cloth, ball, figurine, towel	Distracts person. Keeps hands occupied. Helps person feel more secure
Fear	Have person hold grab bars, tub, or seat	During transfer, person may grab because of fear of falling; helps person feel more secure
	Provide more support, both verbal and physical (e.g., another caregiver) during transfers	Grabbing may reflect the person's fear and need for security
	Involve physical therapy/occupational therapy to determine best method for transfer	PT/OT can provide transfer techniques and training
	Try a different kind of bath (e.g., in-room bath, or shower instead of a tub bath)	Avoids transfers or lifting, which may have made the person fearful
Control	Consider letting person hold onto object you are trying to remove. Be flexible and stay calm	It is OK for person to hold onto clothing, towels, or other personal items
	Have the person help (e.g., wash face)	Keeps hands occupied. May give person a sense of control
Doesn't want to bathe	Come back another time	Respects choice
Interpersonal/Relationship		
Doesn't understand what is happening	Explain each step. Match communication to abilities	Improves understanding; builds trust
Your pacing varies from person to person	Pace your approach to his/her pace	Moving too fast can overwhelm the person
Physical Environment		
Ill-fitting shower chair creates discomfort	Purchase a short chair for a small person, or put a stool under the person's feet	Helps person feel more supported and secure

TABLE 5.14 Tips for When the Person Hollers or Screams

Possible Reason	Action	Explanation
Personal		
Pain	Stop what you are doing and assess what may be causing the pain or discomfort	Helps alleviate source of pain
	Apologize	Helps person feel understood
	Try a different type of bath	A bed bath may be less painful
	Use a very gentle touch	Skin may be very sensitive
	Try a baby washcloth	Softer, will cause less pain
Fear	Warn the person of upcoming sensations by gently touching area and telling person what you are going to do	Eliminates frightening surprises
	Reduce water pressure or use a different way to rinse person	Water spray can frighten person
	Try music. Have the person or family choose a favorite song or tape to play	Can be soothing and can help the person relax
	Sing with the person	Can be soothing and distracting
	Reduce the number of people present	"Strangers" may pose a threat
	Converse with the person	Helps relax and distract. May stop yelling to answer
Control	Give choices	Gives person a sense of control
	Converse with the person about favorite topics	Helps person feel understood, valued
Cold	Put warm water on washcloth	Reduces discomfort of cold cloth
Interpersonal/Relationship		
Doesn't feel understood	Respond with concern each time the person hollers	Helps person feel understood and helps build relationship
Physical Environment		
Uncomfortable equipment	Adapt equipment to the person	Equipment may be painful and may cause yelling
Noisy environment	Try bathing in a quieter environment	Noise may be upsetting

TABLE 5.15 Tips for When the Person Hits, Kicks, or Slaps During Bath

Possible Reason	Action	Explanation
Personal		
Desire for control	Encourage person to help, if possible, with the bath Often this works well when washing the genital/rectal areas or painful areas	Since person may be feeling assaulted, getting person involved allows her to feel a sense of control over what is happening. More dignified
	Say firmly that the behavior is unacceptable, such as "that hurts" or "stop kicking"	Lets person know the behavior is not OK and should stop
	Try the good-guy/bad-guy approach: Assign one person to bathe and another to hold the person's hands gently while talking with the person	This method gets a very unpleasant task done quickly and protects caregivers from harm. Should be used only as a last resort
	Give choices, ask permission	Helps person feel more in control
Pain	Stop what you are doing	Gives opportunity to assess what may be causing the aggression
	Apologize	Helps person feel more understood
	Explore giving pain medication prior to bathing	Older persons have many potential sources of pain related to bathing. Agitation and aggression are often precipitated by pain
Fear	Give person something to hold such as cloth, soap, or someone's hands. Use interesting objects (color and texture, side of shower, chair, towel)	Gives person's hands something else to do. Distracts person
	Call person's name firmly and directly, without yelling	Person will stop and listen
	Reassure person that you're not trying to hurt her	Helps alleviate fear
	Learn defensive self-protection techniques such as blocking blows	Protect yourself from harm
Interpersonal/Relationship		
Doesn't understand what is happening	Slow down or stop: Ask what is wrong	Lets person know you see her as a person, not a task to be done
	Apologize repeatedly and sincerely. Attempt to remedy complaints	Respects person. Helps person feel understood
Physical Environment		
Uncomfortable surrounding	Check comfort of seating device, temperature of water, and room noise level	Problems in these areas can cause aggression
Organizational Environment		
No flexibility in time or form of bathing	Slow down, stop, ask what is wrong, make more comfortable. Discuss with RN or other staff the need for flexibility in the future	Person will feel respected. Organization will be more responsive

TABLE 5.16 Tips for When the Person Bites

Possible Reason	Action	Explanation
Personal		
Fear	Reassure	Decreases anxiety
	Engage person in singing or humming	Keeps person's mouth busy with other activity; distracts
Pain	Explore giving pain meds before you start	Pain is often related to aggression
Hunger	Give person gum to chew or other item such as cookies or beverage (e.g., water)	Keeps person's mouth busy with other activity. Helps alleviate hunger
	Bathe after eating	Prevention is the key
Interpersonal/Relationship		
Doesn't understand/can't inhibit behavior	Beware of mouth if person has a history of biting	Prevent self from getting hurt
	Offer alternatives during bite like gum, candy	Keeps person's mouth busy
	Identify mildly agitated behaviors that occur before biting and take action or back off at that point	Person may bite when very agitated. Try to prevent person from reaching that point
	If person has dentures, don't put them in until after bath, unless person objects	Won't hurt as much!

Try a Bed Bath

It has only been in the last 60–80 years that indoor plumbing, bathtubs, and showers have been commonplace, yet people have been getting clean for centuries (see chapter 2 for the history of bathing). History illustrates that there are many ways to get clean. In-bed bathing is one. The bed bath is often a good choice for persons who are frail, nonambulatory, experience pain with transfers, or are fearful of lifts. In addition, persons who are considerably overweight often enjoy the option of a bed bath to avoid the use of lifts and possible embarrassment in the shower. For these individuals it is also sometimes easier to wash skin folds when the person is lying flat in bed. The bed bath is usually done with a basin of water, soap, and washcloths, and it requires rinsing off the soap. A variation on this method is the covered massage bed bath. Here the person is covered with a large, warm, moist towel containing a no-rinse soap solution. The person is washed and massaged through the towel. The person is warm and covered throughout the bath. It is easily adapted to meet individual preferences. Instructions for the covered massage bed bath are in Table 5.17. Suggestions for individualizing this type of bed bath are in Table 5.18.

It is possible to wash people adequately in bed, and it is often much less stressful. However, there is a belief that people need to be doused or dunked to get clean. In some cases the person's skin actually improves (e.g., less dryness and flaking) when the no-rinse soap method is used in place of a shower. If you have concerns about using a no-rinse method, look for evidence of problems before assuming that a water rinse is necessary. See chapter 8 for a discussion of skin care.

Caregiver Wisdom

With very sick residents, I try the covered massage bed bath. If the person feels bad and can't move very well, it can be more comfortable than a shower. I keep the lights low, talk very quietly, and move slowly. If they seem to hurt, I try to reassure them.

Jose Hernandez, Vencor, Raleigh, NC

When You Think You Have Tried Everything

Sometimes traditional bathing methods, including the covered massage bed bath, just don't work. This presents you with a challenge and an opportunity to use your ingenuity and special caregiving skills. Here are some examples of creative and unique bathing solutions that caregivers have shared:

The Recliner Bath

Several home health aides have reported giving successful baths when the person is resting in the recliner chair in the living room. The aides used a basin of water (preferably with a no-rinse soap) and padded each body part being washed with a towel and incontinence pad if available. This worked particularly well for persons fatigued by chronic or terminal illnesses. If the visits are being covered under Medicare, it is important for the aide to "count" this as a bath for reimbursement purposes. The goal of a bath or shower is to get someone clean and to help the person feel refreshed. This can be done in many ways.

The Commode Bath

This method was useful for a nursing home resident who was easily agitated. Mrs. Harrington disliked being moved or touched and fought through our attempts to carefully shower her or bathe her in bed. She was often incontinent of stool during her morning shower or bath. So the caregiver, Marie, placed her on the toilet in her bathroom, allowed her private time to have a bowel movement, then washed and dressed her upper torso while she sat on the toilet. Next Marie washed her legs and had her stand so she could wash her perineal area and bottom. Her thin hair was washed at the bathroom sink using washcloths to wet and rinse her hair. Marie then transferred Mrs. Harrington to her wheelchair, and she was ready for the day. Some might label it undignified to bathe a person while sitting on the toilet, but for Mrs. Harrington, it was the best way to honor her preferences, needs, and abilities.

The Singing Bath

For another complex person, we tried the singing, sitting, in-room bath. Miss Florence was infamous for refusing her shower and for fighting when she was forced to shower. Estelle, the nursing assistant who worked with her, discovered that she liked to sing, and her favorite tunes were "Jesus Loves Me" and "Happy Birthday." If Estelle waited until she felt Miss Florence was in a good mood, sang with her, performed part of the bath while

TABLE 5.17 The Covered Massage Bath: A Gentle Bed Bath Method

Equipment

- 2 or more bath blankets
- 1 large plastic bag containing:
  - 1 large (5'6" × 3') lightweight towel (fan folded)
  - 1 lightweight standard bath towel
  - 2 or more washcloths
- 2–3 quart plastic pitcher filled with water (approximately 105–110° Fahrenheit), to which you have added:
- 1/2 ounce of a no-rinse soap product (such as Septi-Soft; use manufacturer's instructions for dilution)

Preparing the Person

Briefly explain the bath. Make the room quiet or play soft music. Dim the lights if this calms the person. Assure privacy. Wash your hands. If necessary, work one bath blanket under the person, to protect the linen and provide warmth. Undress the person, keeping her covered with bed linen or the second bath blanket. You may also protect the covering linen by folding it at the end of the bed.

Preparing the Bath

Pour the soapy water into the plastic bag and work the solution into the towels and washcloths until they are uniformly damp but not soggy. They should feel like a well-wrung-out washcloth. If necessary, wring out excess solution through the open end of the bag into the sink. Twist the top of the bag closed to retain heat. Take the plastic bag containing the warm towels and washcloths to the bedside.

Bathing and Massaging the Person

Expose the person's feet and lower legs and immediately cover the area with the warm, moist towel. Then gently and gradually uncover the person while simultaneously unfolding the wet towel to recover the person. Place the covers at the end of the bed. Start washing at the part of the body that is least distressing to the person. For example, start at the feet and cleanse the body in an upward direction by massaging gently through the towel. You may wish to place a bath blanket over the towel to help hold in the warmth. Wash the backs of the legs by bending the person's knee and going underneath. Bathe the face, neck, and ears with one of the washcloths. You may also hand a washcloth to the person and encourage him/her to wash her own face. Turn the person to one side and place the smaller warm towel from the plastic bag on the back, washing in a similar manner, being sure that the person's front remains covered with the bath blanket or warm, moist towel. After washing the back and rectum (with a separate washcloth) remove the back towel and reposition so the person is flat in bed. Use a washcloth from the plastic bag to wash the genital areas. Gloves should be worn when washing these areas. Remove the damp towel before you wash the back or when you're done with the towel bath, depending on the person's wishes and tolerance. No rinsing or drying is required.

After the Bath

If desired, have the person remain unclothed and covered with the bath blanket and bed linen, dressing at a later time. A dry cotton bath blanket (warmed if possible) placed next to the skin and tucked close provides comfort and warmth. Place used linen back into the plastic bag; tie the bag and place in a hamper.

TABLE 5.18 Individualizing the Covered Massage Bath

Change	Explanation
Cover the moist towel with one or two dry bath blankets.	This helps keep the wet towel warm. For persons who are particularly sensitive to cold, two dry bath blankets increase comfort.
Remove the towel before turning the person over to do his or her back.	Some people are more sensitive to cold than others. The wet towel feels cold to them after about 5 minutes.
Do not use a moist towel. Cover the person with a large dry towel and wash under the towel with the four washcloths wet with the no-rinse soap mixture.	Some people do not like the wet towel. It feels heavy or "too wet" to them.
Stand to wash back, genital/rectal area, and rectum.	Some persons feel pain when they are being rolled over. Having the person stand saves a painful extra movement. The person will be getting up to get dressed. The key here is to keep the person covered. This can be done with a dry bath blanket or towel.
Double bag towels with the no-rinse soap mixture.	If the plastic is thin, use two bags; this will help hold in the heat.
Moisten disposable wipes with warm water to wash rectum if it is very soiled.	Wipes tend to be softer and easier to use than a washcloth. The key is to have them warm.
Adjust the light to fit the person's preference (e.g., dim or bright).	Some persons are more relaxed if the lights are low because there is less stimuli. Also, soft lighting and a quiet tone of voice can have a calming effect on the person.

she was lying in bed and part of the bath as she began to get out of bed (following Miss Florence's lead), she was able to wash her entire body. Her hair was done using an in-bed basin on another day. Interestingly, the family reported that Miss Florence had been refusing to get in the shower or tub for 10 years prior to coming into the care facility.

The Waltzing Bath

Mrs. Parker loved shopping and dancing, but she hated her shower. Any time staff tried to get her into the shower room, she became resistive and then combative if they persisted. Her nursing assistants came up with an excellent and creative alternative. They placed numerous washcloths in a plastic bag with a warm solution of no-rinse soap. They removed Mrs. Parker's clothes and covered her with an available poncho-type garment (a bath blanket pinned around the shoulders could also work). One assistant stood in front and began waltzing with Mrs. Parker and talking about shopping while the other was behind reaching under the cover and washing with the warm, wet, no-rinse washcloths. It was quick and joyful for all.

The 7-Day Bath

Family members reported a successful approach to keeping their father, Mr. Simmons, clean by dividing his body into seven parts and carefully washing one each day. He disliked bathing or washing but could tolerate short episodes better than longer, more overwhelming ones.

The Under-the-Clothes Bath

Mrs. Diaz disliked the shower and tub, but she did well when encouraged to wash herself in her room. However, one day her caregiver, Margaret, arrived to find that Mrs. Diaz had been up all night, which was unusual because she preferred to stay in bed most mornings. She was dressed and sitting in her wheelchair. She had a body odor associated with perspiration and urination. A urinary tract infection was suspected and later confirmed and treated. Mrs. Diaz wasn't able to wash herself so Margaret thought she would try to freshen her up and help her feel better. As she talked to Mrs. Diaz about her favorite subjects, she reached under her dress to wash her underarms, breast areas, and genitals. The caregiver had Mrs. Diaz stand briefly so she could wash her rectum. Anytime Mrs. Diaz started to become angry or upset, Margaret stopped to give her time to calm down.

It wasn't a complete bath, but the priority areas were cleaned and Margaret avoided a big battle. Sometimes if a person refuses to remove clothing or holds onto it, you can begin the bath or shower with it on. Often once it is wet, the person is glad to have it removed.

The Shared Shower

Mr. Trask was recently admitted to an assisted living facility. Any attempts by staff to get him to shower or bathe were met with fierce resistance. Instead of forcing him to bathe, the facility called his wife to find out how she had bathed him at home. Mrs. Trask said that she had showered with him and that it had been enjoyable for them both. The wife was invited to shower with her husband at the facility, with the staff assuring privacy. She was glad to be involved in his care and to be able to continue this part of their relationship (M. Calkins, personal communication, November, 2000).

There are an infinite number of ways to keep someone clean without a battle. However, many of the methods described are done outside of a shower or tub, without running water. This means that the hair must also be washed in creative ways.

Creative Hair Washing Techniques

Many persons with dementia resist and fear getting their hair washed. The reasons for this are varied. The most common way caregivers are trained to bathe someone is to start at the top with the hair and work down, working from the "cleanest to the dirtiest" parts. This can cause fearful, angry, and agitated behaviors. It can be overwhelming to have soapy water running into your eyes while you are cold, naked, and vulnerable. You have to wonder about the wisdom of teaching people to start the bath with the most distressing activity.

Caregiver Wisdom

You have to choose the right shower chair. If the one you have doesn't fit the person, you adapt it. You can pad the seat with wash clothes to make it softer. You can use a kid's padded potty seat insert available at stores for about $10 to make the hole smaller and the seat more comfortable.

Kathy House, Fairlawn Good Samaritan Health Center, Gresham, OR

It's helpful to think about why, when, and how to wash hair.

- **Why:** The goal of hair washing is to clean the person's hair in pleasant or at least tolerable ways.
- **When:** Wash hair only when it is dirty if the person doesn't enjoy it. Waiting until the end of the shower to wash the hair works best with most individuals. Often it is necessary to separate hair washing from the rest of the bath.
- **How:** Cover the person with dry towels or a bath blanket. Then try one of the following methods:

> *Wet washcloth method.* Sometimes simply wetting and rinsing the hair using wet washcloths is useful. It is surprising how little water is required to adequately cleanse the hair. This technique works well for washing the hair outside of the shower room also. For example, you could use the basin and washcloth method with the person fully clothed by protecting the clothes with plastic and a towel on the shoulders.
>
> *Beauty parlor sink method.* Going to the beauty parlor has been a pleasant, routine experience for many women. Continuing this activity as long as possible is certainly desirable for reasons of familiarity, enhancing the person's physical appearance, and socialization. You can use the sink in the beauty parlor when no one else is there. It's comfortable, convenient, and familiar to many.
>
> *In-bed inflatable basin method.* Washing the hair in bed with a soft, plastic, inflatable basin with a drainage tube (see Figure 5.1) can be very simple and soothing. Place the person's head in the opening padded with washcloths to make it warmer and softer. Pour water from a pitcher onto the hair. Avoid drops on the face or in the ears as this can cause distress. A good time for this is early morning or after a nap.
>
> *Dry or no-rinse shampoo method.* There are a number of products that allow you to wash hair without using water. Some are powderlike substances and some are a liquid you rub into the hair and towel dry off. If you are using a liquid, it is helpful to warm it to body temperature before applying. Placing the bottle in a microwave or warm water will achieve the desired temperature. There is also a disposable product similar to a shower cap with no-rinse shampoo and

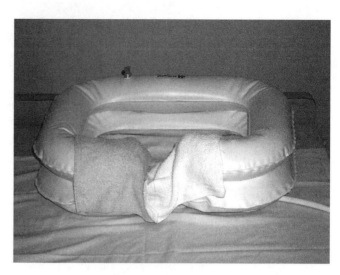

FIGURE 5.1   Inflatable basin.

conditioner that is heated in the microwave and placed on the person's head. The head is then gently massaged for 2–3 minutes and the cap removed. These no-rinse hair products can be useful as interim steps, but eventually the hair may require a more thorough rinsing.

Jelly-in-the-hair. When all your efforts fail you have to find a way to maintain both the person's appearance and right to say "no." Try finding a reason that the person will accept. One caregiver used "jelly-in-the-hair" as a last resort. Mrs. Trent adamantly refused to let anyone wash her hair in spite of repeated attempts and approaches. She would bathe but not let any water near her head. After many weeks of alternative methods, it was clear something else needed to be done. This facility subscribed to the philosophy of getting people to "yes" rather than forcing them to do something against their will. Georgia, a nursing assistant, had an idea. At breakfast, she "tripped" so the toast landed jelly side down on Mrs. Trent's head. After apologizing and "cleaning" it off with a dry napkin, the woman could feel that her hair was still very sticky. Georgia asked her to come to the sink (hair washing sink) so she could try to get the jelly out. Georgia was able to step-by-step add a little more water. Finally she got Mrs. Trent to agree to have her hair washed (M. Calkins, personal communication, November 2000).

Caregiver Wisdom

Finding a reason can really make a difference. You can't force anyone! One person who hates a shower will take a bath if I catch her in a good mood and then talk about her husband. I say: "He likes it when you smell so good!" Then when we're in the shower I make her feel special because she likes to be waited on.

Angell Neal, Brian Center of Clayton, Clayton, NC

The Very Last Resort

Sometimes you can do your best, be creative, wait, try different approaches and still fail to get the person to "yes." These instances will be very rare if you apply the principles of problem solving described here. There may be situations where there is a compelling health reason requiring you to go ahead with bathing in spite of protests. For example, when you are confronted with a person who has been sitting in a large, incontinent, loose stool that is now getting all over, you need to do something quickly to prevent skin irritation and infection. Often in these situations, there may be some acute illness that is making the person uncomfortable and irritable. This needs further evaluation, but in the meantime you need to do something.

As a last resort, try the "good guy-bad guy" approach. Here you and another caregiver should carefully plan how you will bathe the person and have all supplies and equipment ready so it can be completed quickly and efficiently. One person talks to the person and loosely holds the hands to prevent him from striking you or the other staff member. This caregiver apologizes profusely to the person telling him that you understand that he doesn't like this and is angry or afraid. You reassure the individual that it will be over soon. The second person is efficiently but gently washing and cleaning the person. After the task is done it is important to debrief with the person, again apologizing. Doing something to soothe or bring pleasure to him (e.g., providing a gentle backrub or cup of coffee) is a good thing to try, but often a person would prefer that you just get out of his sight!

Again, this approach should be reserved only for situations where there is a compelling health reason to bathe the individual against his will. Body odor without an underlying infection or skin breakdown is not a compelling reason. It has social implications but not health ones. Family request is also not a compelling health reason. That requires education and partnering with the family to problem solve. Incontinence of both bowel and bladder can usually be cared for without the need for a full bath or shower, so in and of itself it is not a reason to "have to" put someone in a shower or tub to get him clean. Remember that when you proceed against a person's wishes the person may feel attacked. We can't permit our routine care to support a practice where the care recipients feel they are being attacked for "their own good."

Testing the Solutions

Did you meet your goal? Do additional changes need to be made? The best approach is to return to your original observations on the frequency and possible triggers of the behavioral symptom. Determine the level of improvement. You can photocopy the Intervention Planning Form (Exhibit 5.1) and use it to record your interventions and observations. For example, during your initial observations the person cried every time you tried to wash between his/her toes with a washcloth. You hypothesized that this was due to pain because this person has arthritis. The solutions you chose were to first warn the person that you were going to wash between the toes, helping him/her get ready for the task. Then you used a cotton swab with warm water and soap to clean this area. The person still cried, although the cries were not as loud or as long. The person was quiet when you washed between the big toe and the second toe, but the little toe seemed particularly sensitive. You have made minimal progress toward your goal of meeting his/her need for a reduction in pain during the bath. You measure this lack of pain by a reduction in crying during feet washing. The person is somewhat better. Again, you hypothesize about what is triggering the behavior. It could be that some areas of the feet are more sensitive than others and that you need a different approach.

Now you have to decide if there are other ways to meet your goal. Return to the list of possible solutions for feet washing (Table 5.11). Which one is most likely to reduce continued pain? You decide to separate feet washing from the bath and to try soaking his/her feet in warm water and then washing them gently with a soft cloth. Again, you assess the effect of this new solution and find that he/she only cried once, when you touched the little toe of the right foot. This is good progress toward

EXHIBIT 5.1   Intervention Planning Form

INTERVENTION PLANNING FORM

Today's Date ___/___/___

Instructions: Record interventions and the results for each bath. Use the Bathing Book to help with developing the plan.

Name: _____

Behavioral Symptom	Possible Cause	Goal	Solution	Effectiveness (see coding below)*	Comments (describe behavior)	Plan

* The intervention made the problem: 1 = Worse   2 = Somewhat worse   3 = No change   4 = Somewhat better   5 = Better

Comments: _____

your goal. The person is much better. You can decide to continue soaking the feet prior to washing them and each time assess the success or failure of this option. Keep your Intervention Planning Form in a flow book. It will help other caregivers know what new solutions have been tried, how they have worked, and new ideas to try. Update the form as needed.

SUMMARY

Selecting solutions that fit individual needs and preferences can greatly increase the comfort of bathing for most persons with dementia. There are many different ways to maintain cleanliness. Set realistic goals for the bath and choose solutions based on your knowledge of the person. Observe the person's response and move on to the next step, evaluating the effectiveness of your solution.

We have identified a three-step process that helps you develop a plan to address behavioral symptoms. This involves assessing and understanding the person and the behavior, selecting solutions to try, and then testing solutions to meet individual needs. Your initial plan is just the beginning of the process that requires continual monitoring and readjustment. As cognitive or health status changes occur, you will also need to modify your plan to meet the changing needs of the person.

---

[1] The material in this chapter is adapted with permission from: Rader, J., & Barrick, A. L. (2000). Ways that work: Bathing without a battle, *Alzheimer's Care Quarterly, 1*(4), 35–49.

PART II

Special Concerns

CHAPTER 6

Person-Directed Care: Sustaining Interactions Through Offering the Needed Level of Assistance

Carla Gene Rapp

FACILITATING ACTIVITIES OF DAILY LIVING: SELECTING A LEVEL OF ASSISTANCE

For most of us, getting dressed is a practical activity to get covered, warm, and ready for the day—an activity we do completely independently and also without much thought. For example, we do not think about how we fasten buttons. We may be more conscious of dressing and taking pleasure in it if we are going somewhere special, but, generally, dressing is just a task to be performed. The same is true for bathing, a task necessary to keep skin clean and free from odor, dirt, and germs, but one we rarely think much about. Dressing and bathing are activities commonly done sequentially. Bathing starts with undressing and ends with dressing. While dressing and bathing are usually simple and unconscious activities for people without cognitive or physical limitations, these same tasks are often very frustrating for the caregiver and the person with dementia.

Most persons with dementia have limitations in one or more of four specific areas: (a) attention, (b) language (seen as the inability to follow one-step verbal commands), (c) sequencing, and (d) judgment. These limitations lead to the need to collaborate with a caregiver to be able to complete activities of daily living (ADLs) such as bathing or dressing. Each person's individual limitations can guide you, the caregiver, in deciding how much assistance you should offer to facilitate the completion of the task.

Level of assistance refers to how much help a person needs. It can range from no help at all, to modifying the environment, to giving verbal prompts, to giving some amount of physical guidance. Table 6.1 contains definitions and suggestions for when to use each level of assistance.

Each level of assistance has specific strategies associated with it. Dementia affects persons in a variety of ways over time. Target the strategies you offer based on each individual's needs. Using the appropriate prompts and assistance, caregivers can facilitate the use of preserved skills by persons with dementia, who will then function more independently. Examples of using preserved skills include holding up a coat, and then the person with dementia will put his arms in the sleeves to help put it on, or handing the person with dementia a cup, and then he will raise the cup to his/her mouth and "drink" from it. When caregivers provide too much (or the wrong kind of) assistance, excessive dependence or excess disability occurs. A person with excess disability appears more impaired than he actually is. Usually one cannot determine how much ADL dependence is related to actual physical or cognitive impairment, improper medications, problems in the physical environment, or caregiver beliefs and behaviors (all potential factors in creating excess dependency). Collaborating during ADLs and offering a level of assistance that maximizes the person's strengths and increases his feelings of success can reduce excess dependency.

Caregiver Wisdom

Your approach has to match the person's needs and abilities. You need more than one trick up your sleeve. Plus, how you present yourself when you enter the room makes a difference.

Janine Nelson, CNA, CMA, Providence Benedictine Nursing Center, Mt. Angel, OR

I would like to acknowledge Valorie Shue, BA, and Cornelia Beck, PhD, RN, FAAN, my coauthors on the previous version of this chapter.

TABLE 6.1 Levels of Assistance and When to Use Them

Level of Assistance	Definition	When to Use
ENVIRONMENTAL MODIFICATION:	Altering the environment to cue or encourage an action—for example, closing the door to reduce distractions or laying clothes out in the correct order.	Supports the person who has problems putting things in order, paying attention, and making good decisions. Compensates for these problems by controlling what is around the person.
VERBAL PROMPT:	Asking the person to begin the action or talking him/her through the task.	Supports the person who has trouble starting or following through on a task. When the person cannot tell left from right, give verbal prompts, saying "this," "that," and "the other" instead of "right" or "left." The prompts support the person who has trouble understanding when someone speaks to him/her and who has trouble paying attention. Repeat your prompts if a person processes slowly. Use this strategy with someone who does not understand words at all, but always use it with people who have impaired verbal communication.
MODELING/GESTURING:	Demonstrating or "acting out" the task for the person to imitate or using gestures to start or guide the person through the task.	Supports the person who has trouble speaking or understanding words and paying attention but who can imitate actions. Sometimes modeling/gesturing works better if you also use words (verbal prompts).
PHYSICAL PROMPT:	Touching the person gently to attract her attention or to indicate which part of the body to move.	Supports the person who can both start and continue a task but who has problems understanding words. These prompts refocus the person's attention or help direct his/her actions. Use physical prompts with verbal prompts to better communicate and collaborate with the person.
PHYSICAL GUIDANCE:	Guiding the person through the task by helping her make the body movements necessary to complete the task. When using physical guidance, start the activity for the person, then allow her to complete the activity independently.	Supports the person who cannot start or imitate an action but who can carry through once you start the step. This person usually has problems understanding words when giving help with a task. Guide the person's movements when giving help with a task. Do movements "with" and not "for" the person.
OCCASIONAL PHYSICAL GUIDANCE:	Providing minimal physical guidance only when the person gets distracted or is not responding. The person who requires occasional guidance can start the activity, but at times the person will require your assistance to restart or redirect an action.	Supports the person who can start but cannot continue an activity and who has trouble understanding words. Only give physical guidance when the person stops responding.
COMPLETE PHYSICAL GUIDANCE:	Performing all necessary body movements while guiding the person through the steps of a task.	Supports the person who cannot start, imitate, or continue an action. The person usually has difficulty speaking or understanding words as well.

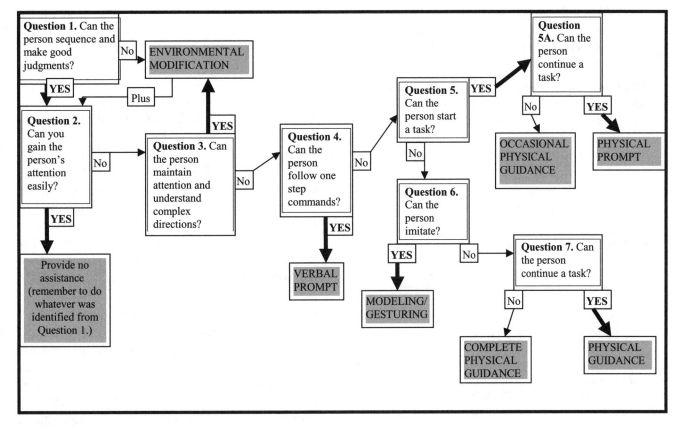

FIGURE 6.1 Level of assistance decision-making guide.

Imagine that this is the first day you are working with Mrs. Jones, a 78-year-old woman who has dementia. Other caregivers have talked about their experiences helping Mrs. Jones get bathed and dressed, saying that she "never helps," that you "need to do everything for her," and that she "always complains about what she is wearing." Upon entering her room, you find her sitting on the side of the bed, looking at her breakfast tray. You notice that her food has not been cut, nor have the sealed containers been opened. You ask if she needs help cutting her food and opening the containers. She replies that she does, and you assist with these tasks. When you finish, she starts eating. Based on this interaction with her, do you believe that Mrs. Jones will need to be completely bathed and dressed? What leads you to this conclusion? How would you plan to collaborate with Mrs. Jones during her bathing and dressing (choosing the specific strategies you would use when working with her)? This chapter will describe a decision-making process that can be used to identify what level of assistance and what specific strategies will sustain interactions and

will facilitate a person with dementia to do as much as possible without help.

Selecting the Needed Level of Assistance

To best facilitate the person's abilities, you must first find out how much help the person needs. The process of deciding the appropriate level of assistance is fairly simple and will be presented both in the text that follows and in Figure 6.1.

The process involves asking a series of questions.

Question 1. Can the person sequence and make good judgments? Difficulty sequencing means the person performs a task with steps in the wrong order (e.g., picks up washcloth, wipes face with it, attempts to apply soap, wets washcloth, puts cloth down). Impaired judgment means the person makes unsuitable decisions (does not try to stay clean or have a neat appearance; wears underclothes on top of shirt or pants). When the person has trouble sequencing or making good judgments, he will need at least ENVIRONMENTAL MODIFICATION. Regardless of your answer here, go to Question 2 (see Figure 6.1).

Question 2. Can you gain the person's attention easily? If you can, the person will notice you when you enter the room or when you speak in a normal tone of voice. If you cannot easily gain the person's attention, the person will ignore you, or you will need to touch the person or speak loudly to get the person's attention. If you cannot gain attention easily, go to Question 3. If you can gain attention easily, then use your answer from Question 1 (whether the person can sequence and make good judgments) to determine the level of assistance:

a. If the answer is yes, the person needs no assistance.
b. If the answer is no, the person needs ENVIRONMENTAL MODIFICATION.

Question 3. Can the person maintain attention and understand complex directions? If yes, the correct level of assistance is ENVIRONMENTAL MODIFICATION to adjust for the person's impairment in sequencing and making good judgments. However, if the person is able to pay attention for only short periods; ignores people, objects, and sounds; and doesn't follow directions that include many steps (e.g., unbutton that shirt, put it on, button it up), a different level of assistance will be needed. Proceed to Question 4.

Question 4. Can the person follow one-step verbal commands? Ask the person to perform a simple task that he should be able to do (e.g., close your eyes). If he can, use VERBAL PROMPT. (Don't forget to review your answer from Question 1 to see if you should use ENVIRONMENTAL MODIFICATION, too.) If the person cannot follow one-step verbal commands, go to Question 5.

Question 5. Can the person start an activity? To find out if the person can start a task, see if the person can use a common object correctly (e.g., lifts cup to mouth) when you put the item in front of (or hand it to) him. If the person can start a task, go to Question 5A. If the person cannot start a task, go to Question 6.

Question 5A. On Question 5, you answered that the person could start a task. Now ask: **Can the person continue that task?** Watch the person while he performs the task (e.g., place the cup in front of the person, touch his hand, and see if he picks up the cup, starts drinking from it, and continues until satisfied). If the person can both start and continue a task, use a PHYSICAL PROMPT since the person has a hard time understanding words. If the person can start a task but forgets to continue the task, he will need OCCASIONAL PHYSICAL GUIDANCE whenever he stops doing the task. (Don't forget to review your answer from Question 1 to see if you should use ENVIRONMENTAL MODIFICATION, too.)

Question 6. Can the person imitate a movement (e.g., clap hands, touch chin)? If the person can imitate, the person needs the level of assistance called MODELING/GESTURING. (Don't forget to review your answer from Question 1 to see if you should use ENVIRONMENTAL MODIFICATION, too.) If the person cannot imitate, ask Question 7.

Question 7. Can the person continue an activity? To do this, start a task and see if the person can complete it (e.g., place the comb in the person's hand and gently guide the person's hand with comb to his head. See if he then combs hair.) When the person can continue a task, he will need PHYSICAL GUIDANCE to start the task but probably can follow through without help. However, if the person cannot continue a task, he will need COMPLETE PHYSICAL GUIDANCE to both start and finish the task. (Don't forget to review your answer from Question 1 to see if you should use ENVIRONMENTAL MODIFICATION, too.)

FACILITATING ACTIVITIES OF DAILY LIVING: STRATEGIES

Level of Assistance Strategies

You have now figured out what level of assistance (how much help) will be most appropriate when working with the person. Each level of assistance has different strategies that you can use when collaborating in ADLs or other care interactions. When facilitating interactions that encourage maximum independence, you will want to use all of the strategies for the chosen level of assistance. In addition, you may use some of the strategies from levels that provide less help. Only in rare cases will you want to use strategies that give more help as they encourage excess dependency. Refer to Table 6.2 for a listing of the specific strategies suggested for each level of assistance and tips on how and when to use them.

TABLE 6.2 How to Provide Assistance at Various Levels

Level of Assistance	Specific Strategy	How and When to Use
ENVIRONMENTAL MODIFICATION:	Use a solid color background that is dark to contrast dressing or bathing items.	Use a dark-colored bedspread as a background when putting out clothes to use in dressing. This strategy helps the person who cannot tell shades, colors, or patterns apart.
	Arrange items in the position and order in which the person will use them.	Arrange clothes face down in a pile on the bed from bottom to top in the appropriate order for dressing with the first item on the top of the pile and the last item on the bottom. This strategy helps the person with sequencing problems.
	Hand items in the correct position.	Hand a brush with the handle facing the person so the person can start brushing her hair without having to turn it around first. This strategy also works well with putting items in the correct order and position.
	Place item(s) beside the part of the body that the person will use to finish the task.	Cue the person to put on the shoes by placing each shoe by the correct foot. For this strategy to work, the person must be able to see the item when you place it by the part of the body and move well enough to start the task.
	Reduce number of options available (let person choose from only two options).	Allow some control when putting on lipstick. Limit choices to one red and one pink instead of offering 10 lipsticks. This strategy helps when the person has poor judgment or wants control (especially when the person complains or changes clothes if she dislikes the clothes you have chosen or refuses to use items that you offer).
VERBAL PROMPT:	Introduce ADL items one at a time.	Say the name of each item (washcloth, soap, towel) as the person picks it up or as you hand each item to her. Saying the name of each item may help the person correctly recognize it.
	Provide brief, simple verbal directions.	Use this strategy by saying, "Mrs. Brown, pick up the shirt." (pause) "Put your arm in the sleeve, pull the shirt around your back, and put your other arm in the other sleeve." (pause) "Pull the front closed and fasten the buttons." The person may need verbal prompts every so often or the whole time.
	Repeat your verbal prompt.	Some people can respond to verbal prompts but may need extra time to process (i.e., time for the brain to figure out what the body is supposed to do). To increase the amount of processing time, count to 10 before repeating the prompt.

(continued)

TABLE 6.2 (*continued*)

Level of Assistance	Specific Strategy	How and When to Use
MODELING/GESTURING:	Show the person what to do (point to the item that the person will use, or show the person how to do a step of dressing/bathing by making the right motion for that step yourself).	Point to the toothbrush as a signal for her to pick up the brush. Then act out placing the brush under running water.
PHYSICAL PROMPT:	Use gentle physical touch to show the person which part of the body to use.	Touch the left leg of the person if you want her to lift it. To use both verbal and physical prompts, touch the leg while saying, "Lift this leg." This strategy also helps get the person's attention.
PHYSICAL GUIDANCE:	Use physical guidance to start the person's movement, then allow the person to complete the action without help.	Place the washcloth in the person's hand, guiding the hand to the water to get the washcloth wet. Guide the washcloth to a soaped area of skin. The person then rinses off the soap.
OCCASIONAL PHYSICAL GUIDANCE:	Provide minimal physical guidance to restart a task only until the person resumes the task without help.	When the person stops washing her arm, move her hand in a washing motion until she resumes washing independently.
COMPLETE PHYSICAL GUIDANCE:	Perform all body movements while guiding the person through the steps of a task.	Lift the person's arm and guide it through the sleeve of the shirt, then lift the other arm and guide it through the other sleeve. Guide her hands to pull the shirt closed in the front and into the correct position.
	Use reverse chaining (graduated physical guidance) by allowing the person to finish the step, and decrease help as the person is able to do more.	On day one, assist the person as outlined above. On day two, provide complete physical guidance until it is time to pull the shirt into the correct position. At this point, stop helping to see if the person will complete the task. Continue doing less and less physical guidance as the person performs more independently. This strategy works best when the person can finish a task but is unable to start it.

Caregiver Wisdom

I try to set it up so it is easy for them. As a person begins to lose skills as part of the dementia, you have to continually adjust. You want to maintain the person's abilities, but if she becomes too frustrated, you want to offer assistance in a way that allows the person to maintain dignity.

Beth Parker, Marian Estates, Sublimity, OR

Standard Strategies

Use the standard strategies (Table 6.3) with each person who needs assistance.

The first two strategies (one-step commands and verbal praise) clearly apply when the person can understand words; however, even when the person generally does not understand words, these strategies create a calm and respectful atmosphere. Also, there is a chance that the person will understand the meaning or intent if not the words. The next two standard strategies require individualization (choosing appropriate/desired reinforcers and identifying the best way to structure the activity) but should apply to anyone with dementia. The final strategy (anticipating the need for help) requires that you select the needed level of assistance strategies for the specific person. When you determine the kind and amount of help the person needs, and at what point the person needs this help, the two of you can collaborate. Overall, the standard strategies are a way to make the level of assistance strategies work better.

CONCLUSION

Using the decision-making process presented in this chapter, you can facilitate interactions that will result in increased ADL independence for persons with dementia. The core of this process is considering each person's specific strengths and weaknesses. No strategy will work with every person, and the person's response will vary from day to day. This makes working with the person a daily challenge. However, the decision-making process described in this chapter is one way to improve the quality of life and care of these persons. The case study in the appendix of this chapter illustrates how this decision-making process can be used. The process described here

will work equally well in acute-care hospitals, private homes, assisted living, or nursing homes. Through use of these strategies, caregivers can facilitate interactions where these persons can perform their activities of daily living as independently as possible.

APPENDIX

Case Study

Mrs. Brown, an 84-year-old white female, has dementia, hypertension, and Parkinson's disease. When she gets ready in the morning she often does activities in the wrong order (e.g., tries to wash with a washcloth that is neither wet nor has soap on it) and insists on wearing a short-sleeve shirt without a jacket, no matter how cold the weather. To get Mrs. Brown's attention, you have to be right in front of her and touch her so she will look at you. Even if you can gain her attention, it usually wanders after a minute or two; usually she walks away as well. She rarely speaks and appears to understand what you say to her only part of the time. Mrs. Brown rarely starts a task without help, but she will imitate the movements you make such as mimicking picking up a pair of pants from the bed.

Today you are going to be working with Mrs. Brown. You want to use the decision-making process described in this chapter to help you decide what level of assistance she needs and then select strategies to use when working with her on the task of dressing. Begin with Figure 6.1 and ask the questions there.

> **Question 1. Can the person sequence or make good judgments?** No, Mrs. Brown cannot sequence or make good judgments. You determine that she will need at least ENVIRONMENTAL MODIFICATION. Now go to the next question.
>
> **Question 2. Can you gain the person's attention easily?** No, it is very hard to gain Mrs. Brown's attention. Go to Question 3.
>
> **Question 3. Can the person maintain attention and understand spoken words?** No, once gained, Mrs. Brown's attention wanders easily, and she has difficulty understanding spoken words. Go to Question 4.
>
> **Question 4. Can the person follow one-step commands?** No, Mrs. Brown does not understand words and therefore cannot follow one-step commands. Go to Question 5.

TABLE 6.3   Standard Strategies: How and When to Use Them

Use one-step commands. Speak simple sentences with as few words as possible.	• Tell Mrs. Davenport each step to perform. "Unbutton your pants." "Unzip your pants." "Pull down your pants." "Sit." • If the person does not understand words, you cannot depend on these commands to work, but they may still be helpful. • One-step commands may not work when used alone, but when used with other strategies, one-step commands may increase the person's independence.
Give verbal praise. Use after completion of each step and dressing/bathing.	• Use after completion of each step and after completing the entire task of dressing/bathing. • Say, "Mrs. Brown, you are doing a great job getting those knots out of your hair." "Look how nice you look . . . you did a great job combing your hair this morning." • Use this strategy with almost everyone except for persons who cannot understand any words or who do not respond to this type of support. • When it is unclear if the person can understand words, use this strategy just in case the person understands the praise. • Use as much praise as possible to encourage the person to take part in dressing or bathing.
Offer specific reinforcement.	• Find out what the person likes, then use these as specific reinforcers. For example: Knowing how much Mr. Thompson loves coffee, allow Mr. Thompson to have an extra cup of coffee when he shaves himself with as little help as possible. • Other examples of reinforcers include candy (may need to use sugar-free), reading a favorite magazine, or going for a walk.
Offer consistent activity structuring.	• Every time, begin the ADL activity with a specified body part, then proceed with the specified body parts in the order that these steps are to be completed. • Also, try having the person dress or bathe specific part(s) of his body, with you doing the rest of the body.
Anticipate the need for help.	• This strategy works with the person who is unaware of her need for help or who is unwilling or unable to ask for help. • For example, since you know that Mrs. B cannot touch her toes, you will put the socks on her feet and pull them up to the point on her leg that she can reach to complete the step. • You may want to wait a period of time (count of 10) before giving help. This gives the person a chance to try to do the task before you help.

Question 5. Can the person start a task? No, Mrs. Brown rarely starts a task alone. Go to Question 6.

Question 6. Can the person imitate? Yes, Mrs. Brown can imitate an action. You now know the level of assistance that Mrs. Brown needs: MODELING/GESTURING. Remember that you also identified ENVIRONMENTAL MODIFICATION in Question 1, so you will want to use these strategies, too.

Next, you will determine which of the specific strategies (from Table 6.2 or the "prescription" form that follows this case study) you should use. When selecting strategies, begin with the strategies (Table 6.2) for the levels of assistance you determined in the decision-making process as demonstrated above. Mrs. Brown's needed levels of assistance are ENVIRONMENTAL MODIFICATION and MODELING/GESTURING, so you will use the strategies for these levels. ENVIRONMENTAL MODIFICATION: Use a solid color background that is dark to contrast dressing or bathing item.

Arrange items in the position and order in which the person will use them. Place item(s) beside the part of the body that the person will use to finish the task. Hand items in the correct position. Reduce the number of options available (let the person choose from only two options). MODELING/GESTURING: Show the person what to do (point to the item the person will use or show the person how to do a step of dressing/bathing by making the right motion for that step yourself).

Then you will consider the remaining level of assistance strategies:

VERBAL PROMPT: Give verbal directions during bathing or dressing. Use this strategy in case she DOES understand the words.

PHYSICAL PROMPT: Use touch to show the person which part of her body you want her to use. Choose this strategy to help Mrs. Brown focus on the task.

PHYSICAL GUIDANCE: No applicable strategies.

OCCASIONAL PHYSICAL GUIDANCE: No applicable strategies.

COMPLETE PHYSICAL GUIDANCE: No applicable strategies.

Next, review the standard strategies (Table 6.3). Expect to use all five of these, and be sure to find a specific reinforcer, such as praise, to strengthen desired behaviors.

Mrs. Brown will benefit from the following strategies.

- Use one-step verbal commands. Keep sentences simple. Use one or two words if possible.
- Praise Mrs. Brown after she finishes each step and after she completes bathing or dressing.

- For dressing, begin with her upper body, then proceed to her lower body.
- Anticipate her need for help.
- Reward her for successful task completion. Mrs. Brown loves ice cream. After checking with the dietitian about this being a permanent plan, give her a small amount as a reward.

As time passes, Mrs. Brown's condition may change, and you will need to use this process again to identify other strategies. The goal in using these strategies when caring for Mrs. Brown is to allow her to become more active in her care and more independent in bathing and dressing.

EXHIBIT 6.1 Individualized ADL "Prescription" Form

_____   _____
Person   Location

Use this "prescription" form to communicate specific strategies to use when assisting persons with dementia during ADL care. Fill in the person's name and location. Then follow these steps:

- Circle or highlight the most appropriate level of assistance required.
- Fill in specific information in the blanks under Standard Strategies.
- Write other modifications to the strategies on this form as needed.

Keep the form somewhere that is accessible to anyone who assists the person with her ADLs.

Level of assistance strategies

*ENVIRONMENTAL MODIFICATION:
Use a solid color background that is dark to contrast dressing or bathing item.
Arrange items in the position and order in which the person will use them.
Place item(s) beside the part of the body that the person will use to finish the task.
Hand items in the correct position.
Reduce number of options available (let the person choose from only two options).

*VERBAL PROMPT:
Introduce ADL items one at a time.
Provide brief, simple verbal directions.
Repeat your verbal prompt.

* MODELING/GESTURING:
Show the person what to do (point to the item that the person will use or show the person how to do a step of dressing/bathing by making the right motion for that step yourself).

* PHYSICAL PROMPT:
Use physical touch to show the person which part of the body to use.

* PHYSICAL GUIDANCE:
Use physical guidance to start the person's movement, then allow the person to complete the action without help.

* OCCASIONAL PHYSICAL GUIDANCE:
Provide minimal physical guidance to restart a task only until the person resumes the task without help.

* COMPLETE PHYSICAL GUIDANCE:
Perform all body movements while guiding the person through the steps of a task.
Use reverse chaining (graduated physical guidance) by allowing the person to finish the step, and decrease help as the person is able to do more.

Standard Strategies

Use one-step commands. Speak simple sentences with as few words as possible.

Give verbal praise. Use after the completion of each step and after completing the entire task of dressing/bathing).

Offer specific reinforcement _____.

At each time that dressing/bathing is done, begin activity with _____
(specify body part), then proceed with _____
(specify body part/s and/or order in which steps are to be completed).

Anticipate the need for help.

Special Concerns

CHAPTER 7

Managing Pain

Karen Amann Talerico, Lois L. Miller

Pain has been identified as a cause of behavioral symptoms that lead to battles during bathing. Bathing provides a lot of chances for pain stimulation because it involves transferring, moving arms and legs, and touching or washing body surfaces. However, the person with dementia is often unable to clearly communicate his pain or ask for relief. Most people with moderate to late-stage dementia will never have the ability to say, "I'd like my pain medication about an hour before I get my bath this morning." They may be left with only nonverbal ways to communicate their pain and discomfort, ways that have often been thought of as resistive or disruptive by caregivers. Such behaviors include pushing the caregiver away, hitting, or yelling. If you are aware that pain may be causing the behaviors, the behaviors become understandable as the person's response to pain.

Older people are more likely to suffer from arthritis, bone and joint disorders, back problems, and many other painful chronic conditions. Table 7.1 lists disorders that frequently lead to chronic pain in nursing home residents. Arthritis and osteoporosis are two of the most common. Untreated chronic pain has been associated with poor quality of life, depression, poor cognitive function, decreased socialization, sleep disturbances, and impaired walking. While many studies have been done with older people in long-term care settings, there is no reason to think that pain issues are different for older people who live in the community.

Even when older people report pain, most studies have identified an alarming trend toward leaving pain untreated in as many as 85% of older people with identified pain and/or pain-causing diagnoses (Ferrell, Ferrell, & Osterweil, 1990). Health care professionals have been found to underestimate the presence and severity of pain by as much as 50%–80%. Older people with dementia are often given less pain medication than cognitively intact older people, even with the same pain-causing

conditions (Horgas & Tsai, 1998; Kaasalainen et al., 1998). Communication impairment has been identified as a major contributing factor to the underassessment and undertreatment of pain in people with advanced dementia.

Undertreatment of pain is often due to the fear of getting addicted to opiate (narcotic) drugs like morphine. These fears are generally without basis in reality and should only be given serious consideration in someone who has a prior documented history of addiction. Even if a person has a history of addiction, he may still need opioid medications to adequately treat pain. Luckily there is much that can be done about pain once it is recognized. However, fears about the use of narcotic medications by older people, their families, caregivers, and health care providers continue to interfere with adequate pain

TABLE 7.1   Frequent Causes of Pain and Discomfort in Older Adults

---

Acute injuries, like falls
Arthritis
Back pain
Cancer and cancer treatments
Constipation and/or cramping from laxative use
Contractures (frozen joints)
Dental problems, like cavities, abscesses, broken or poor fitting dentures
Gastrointestinal (stomach) disorders
Headaches
Neuropathies (nerve pain)—diabetic, alcoholic, or postherpetic (after shingles)
Osteoporosis (bone thinning) and associated problems like stress fractures
Old fracture or injury sites
Pressure ulcers (called decubitus ulcers in past) especially during dressing changes
Urinary tract problems, such as infection or spasms

---

management for many people, especially people with advanced dementia. Failing to adequately treat pain can lead to a host of problems and can make the person with dementia open to worsened health as well as poor quality of life.

PAIN ASSESSMENT TAILORED TO PEOPLE WITH DEMENTIA

What can you do to improve the recognition and treatment of pain in people with dementia? Your first step is to look at whether pain is in fact causing your bathing battle. Because pain is so common in older people, and because many people with dementia will not self-report pain or discomfort, all older people with dementia should be assessed for pain (Herr et al., 2006). A comprehensive assessment should include all of the following areas: information on painful medical conditions, direct questioning about pain/discomfort, pain at the moment, a description of pain, assessment of nonverbal pain signs, and unique individual expressions of pain. Once you get as much of this information as possible, you can develop an person-directed plan to decrease pain stimulation, improve comfort, and turn the bathing battle into a more pleasurable experience for both the person with dementia and you the caregiver.

Information on Painful Medical Conditions

One of the most important things you can do is obtain thorough information about the person's past and current medical problems that could be causing pain, such as arthritis, osteoporosis, old healed fractures, back pain, contractures, cancer, and any other condition that can cause pain (Table 7.1). These sources of pain are not likely to go away as a person's dementia worsens, yet pain becomes more difficult to express in words for the person with dementia. There is no solid evidence to suggest that people with dementia feel pain any differently than you or I do. It is also important to know how the person managed pain in the past, what treatments were effective, especially use of medications, and any values or strong opinions about the use of pain medications. Families can be important allies and sources of information in this information-gathering process (Kovach, Noonan, Schlidt, Reynolds, & Wells, 2006). This information can then be used to develop a pain treatment plan that meets the needs of the individual and also is a chance to educate family about the current standard of

TABLE 7.2   Present Pain Intensity From the McGill Pain Questionnaire

Instructions: Try the McGill Present Pain Intensity Questionnaire (Melzack, 1975) to assess the amount/intensity of pain a person is experiencing. This is the most widely used pain measure in clinical care. Photocopy the form and take it with you when you interview the person. Ask the person: "Are you uncomfortable now?" If the person is experiencing pain and can read, show him the form and say: "Show me how uncomfortable you are now." You may have to try this and explain it several times before the person is able to use it appropriately. People with late-stage dementia may be unable to use this scale. If so you may need to use nonverbal signs of pain (Table 7.3) and the person's unique expression of pain (Table 7.4) to identify pain's presence and then follow the treatment of the person's pain until these individual signs of pain go away and/or the pain no longer interferes in daily life, functional status, and care.

Present Pain Intensity

0	No Pain
1	Mild
2	Discomforting
3	Distressing
4	Horrible
5	Excruciating

Sources: Melzack, R. (1975). The McGill Pain Questionnaire: Major properties and scoring methods. *Pain, 1*, 277–299. (Reprinted by permission of the author, Ronald Melzack, PhD.)

care regarding pain and combat widespread false ideas about addiction and opiate drugs.

Direct Questioning

People with dementia who have a potentially painful condition should be asked directly if they are experiencing pain. We have found success by starting with the question, "Are you uncomfortable now?" Many people with confusion, if able to speak, can answer this simple yes/no question. It is important to know the amount/intensity of pain a person is experiencing so that treatment effectiveness can be assessed. Therefore, it is preferable to use a pain intensity rating scale, if possible. A number of rating scales are available such as the Present Pain Intensity Scale from the McGill Pain Questionnaire (Table 7.2), the most widely used measure in clinical practice (Melzack, 1975). Studies have shown that many older people have the ability to use at least one type of pain rating scale, even those with mild to moderate dementia, and that they prefer to use a scale with word descriptors rather than a scale with only numbers (Ferrell, Ferrell, & Rivera, 1995). Finding a scale that works best for each individual is crucial, rather than using one scale that may only work for some people. You may have to use a particular scale several times before the person is able to use it appropriately. Using the scale that works for the individual person consistently over time to evaluate the course of the pain and its response to the treatment plan is important. The goal of successful pain treatment is to ensure that the pain intensity rating is below 4 on a 0–10 scale or below 3 (distressing) on a 0–5 scale or the equivalent on a word scale. It may not always be possible to get chronic pain down to zero on the rating scale for those people with dementia who can use a scale.

At times, some people have tried to use the FACES pain scale that was developed for children, a scale that uses a series of face drawings meant to represent pain. However, there is little support for its use in people with dementia, and some people perceive the faces are showing emotions like anger. People with dementia may not understand that the faces represent pain. Moreover, few have the cognitive ability to hold in their working memory the idea that a specific face represents pain. To correctly use the FACES scale would then require the person to compare the series of faces to his own body and current pain and then create a verbal answer for the questioner. This complex cognitive task is well beyond the ability of many people with moderate to severe dementia and even some without dementia.

In our recently completed study we found the following approaches most helpful in getting pain information from people with advanced dementia. Using information on painful medical conditions, we asked direct yes or no questions about specific types of pain using the words that the person used in the past. It was important to convey sincerity and to allow adequate time for a response, ideally while touching the part of the body where pain might be. We found that some people with dementia were able to effectively communicate pain once a bond was established with the caregiver. Frequently asking if the person was comfortable or had any "hurts or aches" during care activities, which tend to stimulate or worsen pain, helped also. Very few people with advanced dementia were able to use the pain intensity scale. Therefore, we relied heavily on the nonverbal signs of pain (see Table 7.3) to determine whether pain improved. The most reliable information was obtained when the person asking about pain had an ongoing relationship with the person with dementia. The person asking about pain was able to elicit responses and help interpret unique behaviors that indicated pain. Pain assessment is one area

TABLE 7.3 Nonverbal Signs of Discomfort/Pain
frowning
eyes closing
nose wrinkling
squinting
fidgeting
tearfulness
noisy breathing
crying
grimacing
wincing
moaning
holding body stiffly
pushing caregiver away
hitting
yelling
pinching
high-pitched noises
resisting movement(s)

of dementia care where "knowing the person" becomes very important for adequate assessment and treatment.

Pain at the Moment

The person with dementia may not be able to recall pain during a previous time period, such as yesterday or even an hour ago, because of memory loss. Thus, be sure to monitor pain at the moment as well as over time. You will then have information about pain relief and how effective treatments are for the person. Pain assessments should include a pain description, observation of nonverbal pain behaviors (Table 7.3), improving or worsening factors, AND especially the effect of pain on the person's functional status (how much the person walks and takes care of himself). We found that by treating pain successfully, some people in our study actually improved in their walking and self-care, which many people assumed had declined because their dementia was getting worse.

Pain Descriptors

It is important to try a variety of terms to describe pain to find one that is comfortable for that person. Some older adults may say they have no pain, but then they go on to talk about their discomfort, an aching or burning feeling, or about how uncomfortable they are. Ask about the part of the body that you know has been painful in the past (Talerico et al., 2006). For example, the person might respond negatively to the question, "Are you having any pain?" but respond positively to the question, "Is your back hurting?" or "Is your foot bothering you?," especially when you are placing your hand gently on the body part. It is also important to realize that some older people may have language impairments that make it difficult to accurately identify the body part in pain. For example, in our bathing study we observed a woman who called out, "Ow! Don't touch my arm, it hurts," each time a nurse's aide moved her legs. The nurse's aide would argue that she was not touching her arm because she really wasn't. Careful consultation with the nurse practitioner revealed that this woman had a history of stroke with resulting aphasia (language impairment) that caused her to mix up the names for her limbs. She also had severe diabetes with possible peripheral neuropathy (nerve pain) in her legs. Once the direct caregiver was aware of these conditions, she approached the woman more gently and informed her before moving her legs. This decreased the woman's need to call out about her "arms" or to push away her caregivers so that bathing became more pleasurable. Sometimes it takes patience and determination to find the best pain descriptor for each individual person with dementia. There will be times when the person can't be verbal; you will need to rely on the nonverbal signs of pain.

Assessment of Nonverbal Signs of Pain

Assessment of nonverbal signs of pain can be challenging, especially if you are not familiar with the person. However, there are reliable signals that have shown to be helpful in detecting discomfort across studies (see Table 7.3). The assessment of facial signs of pain, like grimacing, can be more difficult in older people because of wrinkles, oral tardive dyskinesia (repetitive mouth movements sometimes caused by antipsychotic drugs), Parkinson's disease, and decreased clearness of facial expressions in people with end-stage dementia (Asplund, Norberg, Adolfsson, & Waxman, 1991). Thus, facial expression alone should not be used to evaluate the presence of pain. It is also important to realize that often there are not vital sign (blood pressure, pulse, and breathing rate) changes associated with chronic pain, so vital signs should not be used as a nonverbal sign of the presence or absence of pain. Once you have identified a nonverbal sign of pain that is common for a specific person who cannot use a pain scale, use this sign to track his pain over time and how the sign changes with pain treatment. This isn't always easy, and it works best if several caregivers who know the person work together to monitor response to treatment.

Unique Expressions of Pain

People with dementia (and even other people) can have unique expressions of pain, and the person-directed approach recommended in this book is especially needed when it comes to pain assessment (see Table 7.4). One woman's unique pain expression was holding her hand to her forehead whenever she experienced discomfort. Her husband told this to the nursing staff, as it had been her lifelong pattern. This allowed her caregivers to know that when she held her hand to her forehead they should do something to help relieve her discomfort to avoid battling during personal care. Some people with dementia who are experiencing pain may become withdrawn and less willing to get out of bed, others may yell and scream, some may moan, some may increase the amount of pacing, while others may actually laugh. Vocalizations of discomfort such as "Ow!," "Ouch!," or moaning are important indicators that are often dismissed by hurried caregivers. Guarding, flinching, or rubbing body parts are other important individual behaviors that can show pain and the need for pain treatment. Attention to these symptoms when they first present themselves can help the person be more comfortable and can help you protect yourself from injury during bathing.

Table 7.4 gives some examples of individual pain signs that can be used by caregivers to follow how a nonverbal person responds to different pain treatments. It isn't so important that caregivers find one paper tool that works to follow a person's pain over time, but it is important for caregivers to follow a consistent sign of pain in each person to see if the individual treatment plan is working.

Caregiver Wisdom

I know my patients very well and can usually tell if something is wrong. I look at their face for signs of pain such as a frown. Or they might be holding a part of their body. I sit and talk with them then and ask if they're hurting and try to get them to point to where it hurts. If they can't talk they might holler or scream. I get the nurse right away.

Edith Durham, CNA, Brian Center of Clayton, NC

TABLE 7.4 Examples of Possible Individual Pain Expressions in Older People With Advanced Dementia

Type of Expression	Verbal Person	Nonverbal Person
Response to questions about pain or pain intensity scales	Admits to pain, especially when touching painful body part "I'm hurting all over"	No verbal response or inappropriate response When touching painful body part shakes head or makes sound like "uh-uh," withdraws body part
Spontaneous verbalizations of pain	"Ow, owie, ouch, that hurts, stop that"	Rare, occasionally will yell or say "ow, ahh, or no" during movement or care
Facial expression	Grimace, furrowed brow, wincing, crying, or whimpering while telling you it hurts	Grimace, rapid blinking, keeps eyes closed, no smile, crying
Body language	Guarding hips or knees or not moving at all Rubbing or holding body part Flinching from touch or care activity	Guarding, rubbing, or withdrawing painful body part Keeps stiff, resists movement, pulls away from care Holds breath or breathes faster during movement and care
Other nonverbal expressions	Stooped slow gait, limping Restlessness, rocking back and forth	Fast pacing, jerking motion of arms, legs Changes in vocalization pitch and frequency ("dit, dit, dit," to "DIT, DIT, DIT!")

Source: Adapted from Miller, L. L., Talerico, K. A., Rader, J., Swafford, K., Hiatt, S. O., Millar, S. B., et al. (2005). Development of an intervention to reduce pain in older adults with dementia: Successes and challenges. *Alzheimer's Care Quarterly, 6*(2), 154–167.

BEHAVIORAL SYMPTOMS

Many of the behavioral symptoms often seen during bathing such as hitting, pinching, and pushing the caregiver away may be attempts by the person to stop movements that are producing pain. This is where your work as a detective in figuring out whether there is a history of pain, current pain-causing conditions, and assessment of nonverbal pain signs will provide clues as to whether pain is the problem leading to the behaviors. It may be enough to change your approach to the person during bathing as discussed in other chapters of this book. One of the most important strategies we found in our study was to tell the person what was going to happen before beginning to touch the person or start bathing, what we call a timely warning (Talerico et al., 2006). While this may seem like common sense, we found that the time pressure and heavy workloads in many care facilities led the caregiver to rush, resulting in "late warnings" that came after care started. Many of the caregivers were trying to give warnings, but they didn't work because the warnings came after the caregiver had already started touching the person. Simply shifting the timing of the warning from late to early can make a major difference.

Sometimes the only way to be sure that pain is not causing behavioral symptoms is to do a systematic trial of gradually increasing pain management (see Table 7.5) and to monitor the person's response using the pain scale or individual behavior you have identified (Kenefick, Schulman-Green, & McCorkle, 2006; Miller et al., 2005). If behavioral symptoms decrease in response to adequate pain treatment using the Pain Medication Trial Step Ladder then you can safely assume that it was an important cause of the behavioral symptoms for that person (Miller et al.). An adequate pain treatment trial requires that caregivers carefully increase the pain medications in response to the person's response, or at regular periods if it is unclear whether pain is causing the behaviors. One of the most frequent problems with pain trials is that caregivers either don't give enough medication or they fail to try other medications when one doesn't work. That is why Steps 3 and 4 of the Pain Medication Trial Step Ladder are essential. Attending to the cautions in each step is also very important. Side effects can be managed, and something like constipation should never be a reason for stopping pain medication.

Many caregivers in long-term care settings have more experience giving psychiatric medicines than pain medicines, and they may believe that the psychiatric medicines are safer. However, common pain medications often have far fewer side effects than many psychiatric medications, like haloperidol, that are given often to people with dementia who have behavioral symptoms, despite very limited proof of these drugs' effectiveness.

TABLE 7.5 Pain Medication Trial Step Ladder

	Suggested Medication	Cautions
Step 1	Nonnarcotic analgesic, like acetaminophen.	Monitor target pain behaviors. Monitor liver studies, never give more than 4,000 mg/day of acetaminophen. Check for side effects.
Step 2	Add low-dose narcotic drug, like morphine 2.5–5.0 mg, to nonnarcotic drug.	Start low, go slow. Monitor target pain behaviors. Prevent constipation with bowel program. Check for side effects.
Step 3	Continue to increase narcotic.	Monitor target pain behaviors, manage constipation and side effects. Start low, go slow, but go!
Step 4	If Steps 1–3 don't work, try a different narcotic. Repeat Steps 2, 3, and 4 until pain is effectively treated.	

We found in our morning care study that hospice nurses can be a good resource for caregivers who don't have a lot of experience with pain medications. While it can be difficult to know when a person with dementia might die, hospice nurses can also help determine if the person is eligible for hospice services since dementia is usually a fatal illness. Regardless of whether hospice services are indicated, it is appropriate for caregivers to try to minimize the pain people with dementia experience.

CULTURAL AND ETHNIC ISSUES IN PAIN ASSESSMENT

The expression and recognition of pain may vary by culture and ethnicity. Some cultural groups, such as Mexican Americans, Ethiopians, and Japanese, place a strong value on *stoicism*, meaning bearing pain without complaint (Lipson, Dibble, & Minarik, 1996). Even within the American culture there may be regional differences or age groups that have strong beliefs about pain, such as people who live in rural areas or those who grew up during World War I. Some members of these groups strongly value self-reliance or may have negative experiences with veterans becoming addicted to morphine during long months spent in the trenches of World War I. Many groups, such as African Americans, Eritreans, and Japanese Americans, may have strong fears of addiction to pain medications and may require extra support in taking medications (Lipson et al., 1996). Other cultures may encourage the sharing of body sensations, like pain. It is important to take culture and ethnicity into consideration during pain assessment, but individual differences are often more important than broad statements about ethnic differences.

There is troubling and consistent evidence of inadequate assessment and treatment of pain for non-White people (Ezenwa, Ameringer, Ward, & Serlin, 2006). Few of these studies were specific to people with dementia but showed evidence of bias against non-White patients in a variety of health care settings with a variety of types of pain. There was little evidence that these differences were due to income, insurance coverage, or pain reporting (Ezenwa et al., 2006). Knowing how a person's culture or ethnicity may affect his pain experience is important. However, the most important thing is to personalize your assessment and treatment plan to the individual's unique values and needs and be aware of any biases that may have a harmful effect on assessment and care, especially in non-White people with dementia.

INTERVENTIONS TO MINIMIZE PAIN DURING BATHING

Many things can be done to reduce the amount of pain experienced by people with dementia during bathing. These include the way the person is approached and touched, environmental factors, nonmedication pain treatments, and the use of medications. Chapters 3 and 4, describe many ideas for reducing pain. Additional methods specific to reducing pain are described in the following sections.

Nonmedication Treatments

When possible, the best thing to do for pain is to remove the cause. For example, a common problem has been the prescription of multiple laxatives for people with dementia. These medicines are usually thought to be harmless. However, we found that several people in our study were receiving so many laxatives that they were getting up at all hours of the night with cramping and loose stools, including one person who had delirium due to high magnesium levels from milk of magnesia given three times a day. Rather than adding a medication to reduce cramping, we worked with the staff to reduce the laxatives until the person had a normal bowel pattern without cramping. The improvement in several of these people was dramatic. As the people in the study became more comfortable, they became less combative during care. For example, the man with delirium from magnesium toxicity became much less confused, more verbal, and less resistive to care. He was once again able to talk and visit with his family and enjoyed improved quality of life. This was another case where it was thought his decline was due to dementia when in fact it was from treatable factors.

There are several ways to reduce pain without using medications. Remember that some older people (and young ones, too) find a long hot soak in a tub is a good way to relieve pain, especially bone and muscle pain. How many of us have found a nice long soak in the tub helpful in reducing pain after activities like gardening, chopping firewood, or even just sitting in a car for a long time? Some urologists recommend a bath with one-half cup of baking soda added to the water to reduce pain and spasm due to infections and conditions of the bladder. Encouraging an older adult to take a bath to relieve pain may help reduce his reluctance to enter the bath. It is important to allow the person time to relax in the bath and not rush him, especially if the bath is being used to minimize pain. Switching the bath to bedtime may also help with pain management, resulting in a decreased need for sleep medication, or allow lower doses of pain medications to be administered.

Many people find that using a hot or cold pack can reduce pain. For others frequent repositioning or a more supportive wheelchair can improve comfort.

Complementary treatments like acupuncture and massage can help minimize pain in people with chronic pain conditions. These treatments have not been as well-studied as medications, but they show real promise for treating pain. We saw a man who had very severe arthritis—so bad that his hands were all curled up. It was very difficult for his care providers to bathe and dress him because he would become very upset, hit people, and try to stay in bed. A massage therapist began to treat him with gentle massage. Initially the gentle touch was provided for a few minutes at a time. He learned to tolerate touch and trust that she would not hurt him.

Eventually, with the help of some narcotic medications too, his pain became much better managed, his hands opened up, and he stopped fighting his caregivers. The massage had a noticeable impact. His behavior of hitting people began to diminish, and it seemed to his caregivers that he was much more comfortable after his massages. As his pain lessened and the increased ability to open his hands became evident, his ability to move himself in the wheelchair also improved.

Other cultures may add herbs like lavender or mint to a bath to reduce pain and discomfort. While there is limited research on this approach, incorporating certain herbs can make the bath more pleasurable. Many bathing products with herbs are becoming available, especially those made for infants and children, as people recognize their usefulness. The nice thing about nonmedication pain strategies is that they often have few side effects but real benefits for people with dementia.

You will need to experiment to find ways that help relieve pain for an individual person with dementia. Be creative in thinking about how to relieve pain. If you are part of a team of caregivers, make sure that you document what you tried and how you figured out something worked or didn't work. This is where your ability in discovering individual signs of pain can pay off as you use these signs to assess how well the treatments work. It may be helpful to count and track how frequently the nonverbal pain sign occurs before and after a new treatment is tried.

Perhaps most important of all is for care providers to be aware of things they do that cause pain and to avoid certain actions or approaches altogether or perform them very gently to persons with dementia. Washing toes, feet, hair, face, private areas, and armpits is particularly likely to cause pain, as is movement of an arthritic or stiff joint. Be gentle!

Medication Management

Finding just the right dose and schedule of pain medication may be a process of experimentation to achieve the best relief with limited side effects (Kenefick et al., 2006; Miller et al., 2005). We recommend that clinicians rely on the American Geriatrics Society (AGS) guidelines for the treatment of pain in older people (American Geriatrics Society Panel on Persistent Pain in Older Persons, 2002). This article provides guidelines on the state of the art for pain treatment according to experts in the care of older people. Table 7.5, Pain Medication

Trial Step Ladder, was developed based on the AGS guidelines and can be a useful and orderly way to find the best medication treatment for a person with dementia. The guidelines suggest that medications be individually prescribed and increased depending on each person's response and side effects. As with other drugs for older people, the adage "start low and go slow, but go!" (that is, starting a pain medication at a lower than normal dose and increasing it slowly but steadily until the target symptom is lessened or gone) will reduce the risks associated with drug treatments. Make sure, however, that enough pain medicine is given so that the person with dementia can be as comfortable as possible. We know most pain in older people with and without dementia is not treated adequately. Thus, there is a greater chance that not enough medicine will be given rather than too much.

The AGS guidelines recommend starting with a non-narcotic analgesic like acetaminophen, moving to narcotic analgesics if nonnarcotics don't work, and increasing the dose or potency of narcotics until you get satisfactory pain relief (Table 7.5). Medications like aspirin or nonsteroidal anti-inflammatory drugs like ibuprofen often have too high a risk for older people with multiple health problems and should not be used in general (see Table 7.6; Beers, 1997). Most people find that the sedative (sleepiness) effects of narcotic pain medications wear off after a short time. While there is a strong fear among many medical caregivers that narcotic drugs may interfere with breathing, this side effect rarely occurs outside of settings where intravenous narcotics are being given in larger doses, like hospital ICUs. Adjuvant drugs, or drugs used with analgesics, may help reduce pain and allow lower doses of narcotics to be used. Some common adjuvant drugs used in treating chronic pain are antidepressant and anticonvulsant medications, but be careful to avoid those drugs thought to be inappropriate or too dangerous for older people (Table 7.6).

Many people get constipation from narcotic drugs, and the use of a laxative can prevent unnecessary discomfort from these medications. It is so important that preventing and treating constipation are included in both Step 2 and Step 3 of the Pain Medication Trial Step Ladder. Increasing fluid intake is an important part of any constipation prevention program, but it can be a challenge. For many older people with limited mobility, bulking agents like Metamucil can cause uncomfortable bloating and gas. Constipation is rarely a reason to stop pain medication. Work with the person's health care provider to find a bowel program that addresses his individual needs without going too far and causing diarrhea or cramping. You may need to do a systematic trial of laxative medicines to find a specific bowel program that safely prevents constipation. Careful attention to this issue will avoid risking the person's comfort and safety, like the man in our study who experienced diarrhea and delirium from too much laxative.

Some people get relief from pain by using salves or ointments. You might offer to use some ointment to loosen up joints before a bath, or explain to the person that you will provide some extra ointment after a bath. This gives the person something to look forward to and helps the person know that you want to make him more comfortable. However, some people with dementia have a hard time with irritant ointments, like capsaicin, because they have trouble interpreting why their skin is burning. An option for people with mouth pain may be to use over-the-counter gels that contain benzocaine to relieve pain with few side effects. Whatever pain medication is tried, use the same process of finding out how the person communicates pain and use a pain scale or nonverbal signs as discussed earlier in this chapter to monitor how they work for the individual. Try an ointment or salve, monitor how the person responds, and then change the treatment until the person is as comfortable as possible, with minimal side effects.

Timing the Medication

Providing medications on a routine basis (around the clock) is the best way to provide consistent pain relief. The use of regularly scheduled medications prevents high and low levels of medication in the person's system and avoids breakthrough pain. Of course, the person's schedule rather than an institution's schedule should guide the timing of drug administration. An example of a problem with timing was when one resident was woken daily at 6:00 a.m. for pain medication because the day shift wanted the night nurse to give the medicine to make sure it was given before bathing and dressing. The person often refused the medicine because he was too sleepy to understand what was happening. The night nurse, tired of arguing with the person, asked to have the medicine discontinued. Instead the medication time was changed to 8:00 a.m., the time when he usually woke up, and there were no further problems with refusing the medicine.

If the person has only occasional pain with movement, it may be appropriate to provide pain medication

TABLE 7.6 Pain and Related Medications to Avoid on Older People (Beers, 1997)

Trade Name	Generic Name	Reasons to Avoid							
		Ineffective	Physical Dependence	Delirium	Falls	Constipation	Urine Retention	Stomach Problems	Other
Darvocet	Propoxyphene	X	X	X	X	X			Liver problems
Demerol	Meperidine	X	X	X	X	X			
Indocin	Indomethacin			X				X	
Butazolidin	Phenylbutazone			X	X			X	Bone marrow depression leading to blood problems
Elavil	Amitriptyline			X	X	X	X		Psychosis
Sinequan	Doxepin			X	X	X	X		Psychosis
Librium	Chlordiazpoxide		X	X	X	X			
Valium	Diazepam		X	X	X	X			
Miltown	Meprobamate	X	X	X	X	X			
All Barbiturates	Phenobarbitol, Secobarbitol	X	X	X	X	X			Narrow range between therapeutic and toxic dose

30–60 minutes before the bath. This helps minimize the discomfort associated with all the activities required with bathing—undressing, transferring to the bath, getting washed and dried, and finally getting dressed again. Our experience suggests, however, that the use of as-needed (PRN) medications works better in home care settings than in institutional settings, where it can be difficult to coordinate medication administration with bathing times. Poorly timed medication can result in the person not getting sufficient pain relief to make bathing a more comfortable and pleasurable experience.

Medications to Avoid in Older Adults

Certain medications are not recommended for use in older people because of their risk for serious and dangerous effects. Table 7.6 lists pain and some common pain adjuvant medications to avoid, since there are many safer, more effective alternatives (Beers, 1997). A geriatrician or geriatric nurse practitioner can help you choose the safest drugs for the older person you are caring for. At times a pain specialist or pain clinic may be helpful if you are having a hard time treating the pain adequately and managing side effects. Hospice nurses can be an excellent resource for complex pain management issues and may be more available in some settings or areas.

COLLABORATION WITH OTHERS

Some health care providers may need to be convinced that an older person with dementia is having pain. You can do this by keeping track of pain reports, frequency of behaviors, and how they have responded to treatment with heat and simple over-the- counter medications like acetaminophen. You must present this information as data in a confident manner so that you can be an effective advocate for pain treatment. Some nurses have suggested that it is helpful to talk about a "pain crisis" when making calls to providers. This encourages the provider to call back promptly and to recognize that untreated pain really is a crisis to the person who suffers from it.

Family members often have critical information about the person's pain history, usual style of coping with pain, and attempts that have and have not worked in the past to relieve pain. Health care providers can work with family members as allies in making sure that pain is adequately addressed and treated in people with dementia. Ask the family member the following questions:

- How does the person usually express pain?
- Are there medications that have helped the pain in the past?
- Are there pain medications that haven't been helpful in the past?
- Does he, or has he in the past, used heat packs or ointments to help relieve pain?
- Are there any other things we should know about his pain?

If you are the family member of a person with dementia who you think is having pain, create a list before you call the doctor or nurse practitioner. Have the answers to the previous questions ready so that you can give the provider enough information to make useful suggestions. You may want to try using acetaminophen for a few days before you call the provider to see if it makes a difference. Be careful not to give too much acetaminophen, using Table 7.5 as a guideline. Whenever persons with dementia go to a specialist, it is critical that they be accompanied by the person who best knows them and their current issues. Be sure to have the answers to the individual pain assessment questions written down for review. This will help ensure that the visit isn't wasted and that the person with dementia gets the best care possible. You may need to advocate for the person with dementia, and having information helps you stand up for the person effectively. Don't take "no" for an answer if you believe pain is causing the battle with bathing.

CONCLUSION

Pain is a treatable condition, whether you know exactly what is causing it or not. Many options are available to treat pain so the person with dementia has better quality of life and caregivers are not placed at risk of harm. Bathing doesn't have to be a battle when you have the right tools.

REFERENCES

American Geriatrics Society Panel on Persistent Pain in Older Persons. (2002). The management of persistent pain in older persons: AGS panel on chronic pain in older persons. *Journal of the American Geriatrics Society, 50*(6 Suppl.), S205–S224.

Asplund, K., Norberg, A., Adolfsson, R., & Waxman, H. (1991). Facial expressions in severely demented patients—a stimulus response study of four patients with dementia of the Alzheimer type. *International Journal of Geriatric Psychiatry, 6,* 599–606.

Beers, M. (1997). Explicit criteria for determining potentially inappropriate medication use by the elderly: An update. *Archives of Internal Medicine, 157*(14), 1531–1536.

Ezenwa, M. O., Ameringer, S., Ward, S. E., & Serlin, R. C. (2006). Racial and ethnic disparities in pain management in the United States. *Journal of Nursing Scholarship, 38*(3), 225–233.

Ferrell, B. A., Ferrell, B. R., & Osterweil, D. (1990). Pain in the nursing home. *Journal of the American Geriatrics Society, 38*(4), 409–414.

Ferrell, B. A., Ferrell, B. R., & Rivera, L. (1995). Pain in cognitively impaired nursing home patients. *Journal of Pain and Symptom Management, 10*(8), 591–598.

Herr, K., Coyne, P. J., Key, T., Manworren, R., McCaffery, M., Merkel, S., et al. (2006). Pain assessment in the nonverbal patient: Position statement with clinical practice recommendations. *Pain Management Nursing, 7*(2), 44–52.

Horgas, A. L., & Tsai, P. F. (1998). Analgesic drug prescription and use in cognitively impaired nursing home residents [see comments]. *Nursing Research, 47*(4), 235–242.

Kaasalainen, S., Middleton, J., Knezacek, S., Hartley, T., Stewart, N., Ife, C., et al. (1998). Pain and cognitive status. *Journal of Gerontological Nursing, 24*(8), 24–31.

Kenefick, A. L., Schulman-Green, D., & McCorkle, R. (2006). Decision making in pain management: Using the model of sequential trials. *Alzheimer's Care Quarterly, 7*(3), 175–184.

Kovach, C. R., Noonan, P. E., Schlidt, A. M., Reynolds, S., & Wells, T. (2006). The serial trial intervention: An innovative approach to meeting needs of individuals with dementia. *Journal of Gerontological Nursing, 32*(4), 18–27.

Lipson, J., Dibble, S., & Minarik, P. (1996). *Culture and nursing care: A pocket guide.* San Francisco: UCSF Nursing Press.

Melzack, R. (1975). The McGill Pain Questionnaire: Major properties and scoring methods. *Pain, 1,* 277–299.

Miller, L. L., Talerico, K. A., Rader, J., Swafford, K., Hiatt, S. O., Millar, S. B., et al. (2005). Development of an intervention to reduce pain in older adults with dementia: Successes and challenges. *Alzheimer's Care Quarterly, 6*(2), 154–167.

Talerico, K. A., Miller, L. L., Swafford, K., Rader, J., Sloane, P. D., & Hiatt, S. O. (2006). Approaches to reduce and minimize pain in older adults with dementia during morning care. *Alzheimer's Care Quarterly, 7*(3), 163–174.

RELEVANT RESOURCES

Clinical Practice Guidelines on the Management of Persistent Pain in Older Adults from the American Geriatrics Society (American Geriatrics Society, 2002).

Web sites on pain:

Web site of American Pain Society, an interdisciplinary organization. http://www.ampainsoc.org/

Web site of Worldwide Congress on Pain; offers pain library and other services. http://www.pain.com/

Web site of American Academy of Pain Management. Help in finding a pain professional. http://www.aapainmanage.org/

Web site of American Chronic Pain Association self-help group for chronic pain management. http://www.theacpa.org/

Web site of The Mayday Pain Project—has links to many other excellent pain Web sites. Some of the links do not work, but the site is there with some good info. http://www.painandhealth.org/

Web site of American Pain Foundation: Focused on a grassroots "Power Over Pain Campaign," whose overarching purpose is to increase the number of Americans receiving effective pain relief. http://www.painfoundation.org/

CHAPTER 8

Care of the Skin

*Johannah Uriri Glover, Kimberly Horton Hoffman,
LouAnn Rondorf-Klym*

Bathing procedures are critical to personal hygiene and maintaining healthy, intact skin. However, prolonged exposure to water, soap and certain hygiene products, and inadequate washing that leaves debris such as urine/fecal matter can all contribute to breakdown of a person's skin. The risk of infection increases once the skin breaks down, especially in an older person whose immune system is compromised. Bathing procedures can be modified to help maintain the integrity of the skin and to decrease the risk of skin problems and infections. This chapter describes skin problems that may occur in older persons and body areas most vulnerable to these conditions. A procedure for checking the skin and infection control issues related to bathing are described. Finally, recommendations for preventive skin care related to bathing are outlined.

Skin Characteristics

As we age, our skin may become wrinkled, dry, and fragile. Exposed areas such as the elbows, knees, and the bottom of the feet can have rough areas. Some flaking or scaling is normal. Light skin may become yellowish and dark skin ashen in color. Gentle washing of the skin with soap and water is the primary means of removing body substances and other debris from the skin such as urine, feces, and perspiration that can cause odor and irritate the skin. Gentle washing can be equally effective with any bath method (tub bath, shower, and in-bed bath). However, skin problems can occur or worsen not because of the bath method chosen but because of the procedures used during bathing. For example:

- Improper drying may lead to skin tears and/or fungal infections.

- Areas left unwashed may result in skin irritations.
- An allergic reaction to soap products may lead to rash or skin infection.
- Soap product residuals may result in dry and irritated skin.

The six most common skin problems associated with bathing and preventive strategies are summarized in Table 8.1.

Skin Assessment

Persons with dementia may be more susceptible to skin problems if their hygiene is difficult to maintain. As a caregiver, you will need to pay special attention to and closely monitor the person's skin to ensure that skin problems do not develop or are recognized and treated early. To prevent added distress, the best time to look at the skin is during the bath when the person is already undressed. Observe the chest, upper arms, stomach area, underneath the arms, back, inner thighs, groin creases, genital and rectal areas, upper and lower legs, feet, and between the toes for skin problems. Look carefully as you assist the person with washing and drying each part of the body. Become familiar with the person's skin so that you can observe changes before they become serious problems. How often you should check the skin will vary with the person's health and skin condition.

The best procedure is to:

- Wash your hands with soap and warm water and dry your hands.
- Provide for privacy and keep the person warm at all times.

TABLE 8.1 Skin Problems Associated With Bathing

Skin Problems	Definition	Possible Causes	Prevention
Foreign body debris	Dirt, liquid, or food spills, body substances (dried blood, saliva, stool, urine) or dead skin cells between folds of skin	Poor hygiene	Clean body areas adequately after close inspection of skin folds and crevices
Cracking or skin tears, fissures	Skin resembles dried earth; slight cracking appearance may progress to tears in the skin	Soap	Use lubricants and moisturizers. Hemorrhoid preparation (e.g., Preparation H™) is good for rough areas on the soles of the foot, elbows, and ankles
Redness, hyperpigmentation (darker color) or hypopigmentation (lighter color)	Pinkish to bright red or scarlet in color. In darker skin, the skins may appear purple or ashen gray when compared with surrounding skin	Soap, allergies, or infection	Rinse area completely and contact the person's health care provider for treatment of allergies and scabies
Rash, eruptions, or primary skin lesions	Bumps containing fluid; may be intact or weeping and crusting	Infection, allergies, scabies	Contact the person's health care provider for the treatment of allergies and scabies
Moist skin (Maceration)	Skin looks thickened and white with boggy appearance presenting with many breaks in the skin	Body parts not completely dried or sweating	Make sure skin folds are cleansed and dried completely, and apply cornstarch to keep the areas dry
Scaling or flaking	Small, thin dandruff-like flakes of dried or dead skin	Soap	Control humidity in the environment. Use lubricants and moisturizers or hydrogenated vegetable oil (e.g., Eucerin™, Keri Lotion™, light oil, or hydrogenated Crisco™)

- Observe the skin carefully and closely when you are removing the person's clothing.
- Check each body area as you wash the skin.
- Rinse the soap away completely (unless you are using a no-rinse soap substitute solution).
- Inspect skin folds for soap before drying (underneath the arms, breasts, and abdomen; in the groin creases, genital, and rectal areas; between the toes).
- Continue to look closely at the skin and folds as you pat the skin dry.
- Report to the health care provider, charge nurse, or other appropriate person any changes you notice.

Observing the skin of persons who are very private, who dislike having parts of the body touched, or who are getting a towel bath in which the skin is not as exposed may be difficult. In these situations, try examining the skin while assisting the person during toileting. You will need to use your ingenuity and skill to assure that adequate observation occurs and that potential problems are discovered and addressed early.

It may be helpful to use a skin assessment form to document your observations and track improvements during treatment. If the person can give you accurate information about her skin and any problems she is experiencing, consider using a self-report of changes in skin condition (e.g., The Skin Detective Questionnaire, Lob-Corzilius et al., 2004). Self-reports may not always be accurate, therefore an assessment tool, which a caregiver can use to document skin condition, may be more useful in obtaining accurate information. Most skin condition assessment tools used by nurses are useful for evaluating serious skin conditions, such as pressure sores. The Skin

Resident Name_____ Date_____ Time_____a.m./p.m.   No lesions_____

Caregiver Name_____   No debris_____

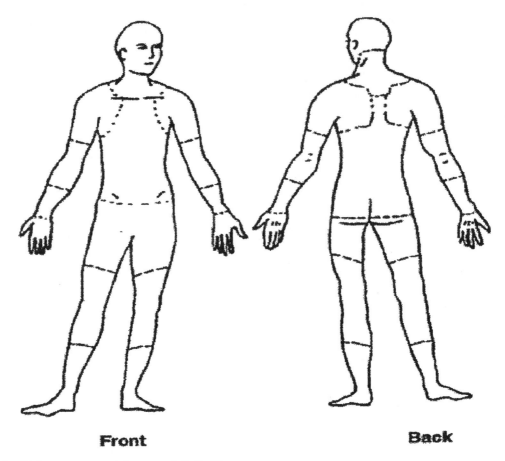

Front   **Back**

FIGURE 8.1   Skin assessment form and definitions.

Comments:

Directions: Assess skin for eight problems. Use the following letters to indicate each problem:
Draw a shape the size of the affected area on the figure. Draw an arrow from the shape to the outside of the figure and label it with the appropriate letter listed below and, if an ulcer, the stage. If no skin lesions and/or debris are noted, check the box in the upper right hand corner of the form.

D = Debris (foreign or body) CODE THIS AFTER BATH	F = Fissures or cracking	R = Redness, hyperpigmentation, or hypopigmentation	Torn or abraded skin
E = Eruptions or primary skin lesions	M = Maceration	S = Scaling or flaking	U = Ulcer

Assessment Form (Figure 8.1) is a tool that caregivers in any setting can easily use to document skin condition. To use this tool, carefully observe the person's skin before the bath. Look for evidence of:

- fissures or cracking
- redness, hyperpigmentation, or hypopigmentation
- torn or abraded skin
- ulcers
- eruptions or lesions
- maceration
- scaling.

If you find any of these skin problems follow these steps:

- Draw a shape the size of the affected area on the figure on the form.
- Draw an arrow from the shape to the outside of the figure and label it with the appropriate letter: E = Eruptions or primary skin lesions; F = Fissures or cracking; M = Maceration; R = Redness, hyperpigmentation, or hypopigmentation; S = Scaling or flaking; T = Torn or abraded skin; U = Ulcer, skin breakage over bony area.
- If no skin lesions are noted, check the box in the upper right hand corner of the form.

Assessing the skin before the bath allows you to determine whether the cleansing agents such as soaps, body washes, etc., used in previous baths are causing skin problems. After the bath, check to be sure the person is clean and no debris or soap residue are left on the skin. If debris is found:

- Draw a shape the size of the affected area on the figure on the form.
- Draw an arrow from the shape to the outside of the figure and label it "D."

Indicate "no debris" on the top of the form if none is found. You can repeat this assessment as often as needed and track progress when changes are made in the bathing routine or products.

Infection Control

Infection control is essential to keep the person's environment free of potential pathogenic microorganisms such as bacteria and fungi that the normal defenses of an older person's body may be less able to fight. Environmental factors such as cross-contamination associated with equipment used during tub baths and showers in shared bathing facilities can contribute to infections. Medications (e.g., antibiotics, immunosuppressants) that change the skin flora contribute to the natural selection of pathogenic organisms. Transient organisms and overgrowth of microflora can become a problem for older adults under these conditions. Thus, basic infection control knowledge is important to prevent infections from occurring and to control infections that are already present.

Caregiver Wisdom

With our residents you have to wash the skin very gently. Make sure you put lotion on it every day, 'cause their skin is so dry. I check for red marks when I do a.m. care and as I dry them after a bath.
     Edith Durham, CNA, Brian Center of Clayton, NC

As a caregiver, you can help prevent the transfer of infection to yourself or others by following these guidelines during bathing activities:

- Keep dirty and clean items separate.
- Replace a clean item that becomes dirty with a new clean item.
- Bathe the person from the "cleanest" areas to the "dirtiest" areas when possible or use different washcloths for different body parts to reduce the spread of microorganisms to cleaner areas of the body.
- Clean bathing areas after each use with a cleaning agent containing chlorine.
- Wear gloves and a waterproof gown when bathing or when providing care if the person has an obvious infection, open wound, or pressure ulcer.

As a caregiver, you can help prevent the growth of microorganisms on the skin by following these guidelines during bathing activities:

- Use tepid water.
- Use a small amount of soap.
- Wash skin gently.

- Rinse soap completely (unless using a no-rinse soap substitute solution).
- Dry skin folds (underneath breast, groin, and axillae) well after the bath.
- Keep skin lubricated.

Know the medications the person is taking and use extra care when the person is taking medications that change the skin flora. Examples of such medications include antibiotics or immunosuppressive drugs.

To prevent and control infections when using a bed bath or basin bath procedure, precautions such as washing hands, using gloves, and protecting clothes with a gown are important also. Generally, wash from the least soiled area to the most soiled area (head, face, neck, upper arms, abdomen, upper and lower legs, and feet). Then, change the washcloth and water (if using a basin) and wash the most soiled areas (genitalia to rectum). If this general approach is distressing to the person it can be safely and skillfully modified to meet personal needs and preferences. For example, different areas of the body can be washed at different times rather than all in the same bath.

APPROACHES TO SKIN CARE TO PREVENT SKIN PROBLEMS

To prevent excessive dryness that may be caused by soap products, the chest, upper arms, upper and lower legs, and abdomen can be washed with a small amount of lotion and water (a couple of squirts of lotion into a basin of warm water). These areas usually are not contaminated with urine, feces, or perspiration. Mild soap such as Dove that contains fats or a gentle no-rinse soap substitute solution that doesn't contain alcohol can be used underneath the arms and in the groin, genital, and rectal areas. These areas need more attention as they are more likely to become contaminated with urine or feces or to trap moisture and organisms that can contribute to odor.

When you are finished washing, be sure that you:

- Rinse off the soap completely unless you are using a no-rinse soap substitute solution.
- Always check the areas for allergic reactions (e.g., redness, swelling, rash) to the cleansing product.
- Pat the skin dry instead of rubbing and apply lubricants after drying the skin.

- Immediately after drying, apply lotion or other lubricants to keep the skin moist.
- To prevent moisture-related problems, check to be sure that the skin folds are dry.

Special products can also be useful. For example, hemorrhoid preparations (Preparation H™ or a generic brand) that include shark liver oil as an ingredient can be used for wrinkles and rough spots or for cracking on the soles of the feet, elbows, knees, and ankles. Avoid lotions whose first ingredient is water and any cleansing product containing alcohol. Choose scented soaps carefully to avoid allergic reactions and increased dryness.

Caregiver Wisdom

I've been a nursing assistant for 7 years. I've learned that if a person doesn't like a shower, you need to try a Keri™ or sponge bath. They smell great and their skin is much better. It's easier to get them clean and you don't need a lot of water.

Terri Johnson, CNA, Hillcrest Convalescent Center, Durham, NC

Ethnic Skin and Hair

Skin type differs among people of different ethnic backgrounds, such as Black, White, Asian, and Latino people. Skin characteristics may also differ. Skin colors range from white, bronze, to very dark. Redness may appear as black or purple in color in persons with very dark skin. Darker skin becomes "ashy" white when the skin is dry and scaly. This may not be apparent in white or very fair-skinned individuals. Many people with dark skin use oils or petroleum jelly to get rid of the ashy appearance.

However, these oils may cause acne. To prevent acne in black skin, products such as lanolin, petroleum jelly, vegetable oils, or waxes should be avoided. Instead, use small amounts of light oil such as olive or fish oils or moisturizing oils such as Keri oil to moisturize black skin and avoid acne.

The hair of individuals with dark skin is often curly, dry, and brittle, causing the hair shaft and scalp to be more delicate and at risk for damage. A lightweight hair oil and scalp conditioner, rather than heavy oils, is recommended for daily care. Furthermore, use shampoos and conditioners made for persons of color. For example, shampoos for curly hair should contain mild detergents, detangling agents, and a pH balance range of 4.5 to 5.5 to avoid damage to the hair shafts from combing and dryness. Since the hair is dry, daily washing is not recommended, but wash hair once or twice a week to prevent scalp dryness.

CONCLUSION

The skin of older adults is fragile and requires special attention and care during bathing to prevent skin breakdown and environments for bacterial or fungal infections. Preventing infection is important especially in an older person whose immune system may be compromised. Moreover, persons with dementia may be at greater risk for these problems. Thus, caregivers in all settings (acute care, long-term care, and at home) need to provide extra care and attention when assisting older persons with bathing. Key points to remember are:

- Check the person's skin routinely during undressing, bathing, and toileting activities.
- Use the skin assessment form to document and track skin condition.
- Select and use soap products that are not irritating to the skin.
- Make sure the skin is clean and dry, especially in skin folds that trap debris and moisture.
- Use moisturizing products liberally to help reduce drying of the skin and breakdown.
- Report any skin changes to a health care provider or supervisor who can assist you in addressing skin problems in older persons for whom you are caring.

Intact skin is a person's first line of defense against irritations and infections. Your attention to a care recipient's skin during bathing will help ensure good hygiene and will help ensure that this barrier—and comfort—are maintained.

REFERENCE

Lob-Corzilius, S., Böer, S., Scheewe, K., Wilke, M., Schon, J., Schulte im Walde, T. L., et al. (2004). The "Skin Detective Questionnaire": A survey tool for self-assessment of patients with atopic dermatitis. First results of its application. *Dermatology and Psychosomatics, 5*, 141–146.

RESOURCES

Brown, D., & Sears, M. (1993). Perineal dermatitis: A conceptual framework. *Ostomy and Wound Management, 39*(7), 20–22.

Finch, M. (2003). Assessment of skin in older people. *Nursing Older People, 15*(2), 29–30.

Fordyce, M. (1999). *Geriatric PEARLS* (pp. 6, 14). Philadelphia: F. A. Davis.

Hardy, M. A. (1990). A pilot study of the diagnosis and treatment of impaired skin integrity: Dry skin in older persons. *Nursing Diagnosis, 1*(2), 57–63.

Hardy, M. A. (2001). Impaired skin integrity: Dry skin. In M. L. Mass, T. Tripp-Reimer, K. C. Buckwalter, M. Titler, M. D. Hardy, & J. P. Specht (Eds.), *Nursing care of older adults* (pp. 137–144). St. Louis, MO: Mosby.

Johnson, B. L., Moy, R. L., & White, G. M. (1998). *Ethnic skin, medical and surgical* (pp. 5, 32–40, 214–217). St. Louis, MO: Mosby.

Kovach, T. (1988). Controlling infection as part of the bath process. *Provider, 14*(12), 43–44.

Leyden, J. J., McGinley, K. J., Norstrom, K. M., & Webster, G. F. (1987). Skin microflora. *The Journal of Investigative Dermatology, 88*(3), 65s–72s.

Lueckenotte, A. G. (1994). *Pocket guide to gerontologic assessment* (pp. 60–81). St. Louis, MO: Mosby.

Mairis, E. (1992). Four senses for a full skin assessment. Observation and assessment of the skin. *Professional Nurse, 7*(6), 376–380.

Montagna, W., Prota, G. P., & Kennedy, J. A. (1993). *Black skin structure and function* (pp. 132–133). San Diego, CA: Academic Press.

Patterson, J. A. K. (1989). *Aging and clinical practice: Skin disorders.* New York: Igaku-Shoin.

Roth, R. R., & James, W. D. (1989). Microbiology of the skin: Resident flora, ecology, infection. *Journal of the American Academy of Dermatology, 20*(3), 367–481.

Sloane, P. D., Hoeffer, B., Mitchell, M., McKenzie, D., Barrick, A. L., Rader, J., et al. (2004). Effect of person-centered showering and the towel bath on bathing-associated aggression, agitation, and discomfort in nursing home residents with dementia: A randomized, controlled trial. *Journal of American Geriatrics Society, 52*, 1795–1804.

Wysocki, A. B., & Bryant, R. A. (1992). Skin. In R. Bryant (Ed.), *Acute and chronic wounds nursing management* (pp. 1–30). St. Louis, MO: Mosby.

CHAPTER 9

Transfer Techniques

Adele Mattinat Spegman, Theresa H. Raudsepp, Jennifer R. Wood

Many people with dementia require assistance getting from their beds to the sink, tub, or shower. For some, support is needed to get out of bed and walk. But for many, bath time encompasses multiple transfers: in and out of bed, to the wheelchair or shower chair, on and off the toilet or commode. While bathing activities provide the benefits of physical activity, bathing also presents risks for injury to both the person with dementia and the person providing assistance.

This chapter describes safe and effective transfer techniques. Therapeutic transfer techniques express respect for the comfort, dignity, and needs of the person with dementia. At the same time, therapeutic transfers protect you from injury. Successful transfers require thoughtful communication skills, good body mechanics, and an awareness of safety. This approach applies to helping a person with dementia bathe as well as to other aspects of providing care.

ISSUES SURROUNDING TRANSFER TECHNIQUES

The most effective transfer technique is one that is directed to the person. It is a prescription for the best means of mobility given the person's abilities. If at all possible, the person-directed transfer should involve some weight-bearing movements. This transfer has several benefits. It promotes muscle strength and range of motion in joints, and improves circulation, maintains bone density, and increases alertness. Osteoporosis is slowed by weight-bearing of the long bones of the arms and legs. Furthermore, active participation in one's care and comfort is linked to increased self-esteem.

The "underarm" method for transfers is popular but can be a risky way of assisting with a transfer (Figures 9.1 and 9.2). For the person being assisted, the underarm

method is a painful way of preventing a fall. It increases the risk of other injuries, such as bruising, muscle strains, nerve trauma, and shoulder dislocation. For you, assisting with a transfer, the underarm method is associated with back injuries and muscle strains. This approach continues to be used, despite the known risks. As caregivers, we must update our practices to provide quality care!

Mechanical lifts are being used to minimize the risk of caregiver injuries. Some long-term care facilities have instituted a "zero-lift" policy so that caregivers do not directly lift residents. Yet the mechanical lifts do not eliminate staff injuries. Most devices also reduce the opportunity for an active weight-bearing transfer. But more importantly, using a lift may be frightening for a person with dementia. The experience may heighten the person's confusion, anxiety, and resistance to the transfer. Unfortunately, we often direct our attention to the mechanical device instead of to the person being transferred. Caregivers were found to communicate less during transfers when mechanical lifts were used in comparison to transfer approaches without a lifting device (Wood, Raudsepp, Miller, & Dazey, 2000). Although lifts are a valuable tool for safe transfers, the use of mechanical devices is not a panacea. Careful consideration of the pros and cons is required in each individual case.

Caregiver Wisdom

Some places I have worked have a no-lift policy. There is a better way. Our techniques are safe for the staff and allow people to use as much of their abilities as possible.
Janine Nelson, CNA, CMA, Providence Benedictine Nursing Center, Mt. Angel, OR

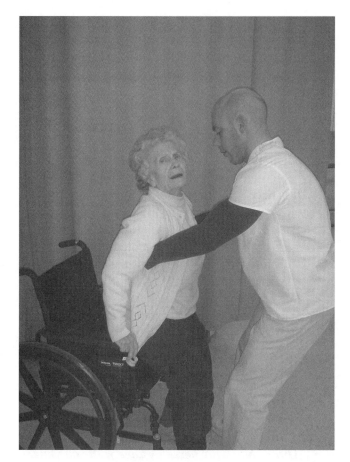

FIGURE 9.1 Incorrect underarm transfer method—one-caregiver assist.

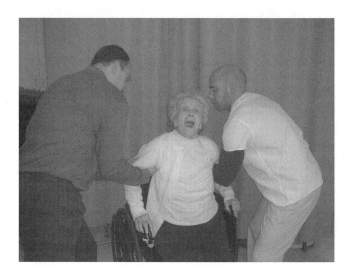

FIGURE 9.2 Incorrect underarm transfer method—two-caregiver assist.

THE BASICS OF SAFE TRANSFERS

Three issues are fundamental to all successful transfer techniques:

- good body mechanics
- attention to safety
- cueing the person being transferred.

Good body mechanics refers to how you position and use your body as well as the position of the person being transferred. Safe techniques require that you know how to use your resources: equipment, other caregivers, and a variety of transfer techniques. Perhaps most important, providing information about the transfer to the person being transferred maximizes participation and decreases anxiety.

THE BASICS OF BODY MECHANICS

Take care of yourself! The job description of a caregiver requires flexibility, strength, and stamina. It has been described as one of the most dangerous professions in America due to the high incidence of back injuries. Good body mechanics is a first defense toward preventing injury (Table 9.1). As caregivers, we are responsible for achieving a fitness level that meets the physical demands of our caregiving activities. Some of the physical demands include:

- tolerance of repeated bending and stooping
- ability to lift 50 pounds while maintaining good body mechanics
- ability to fully squat
- ability to kneel on one or both knees, then rise up without relying on your arms.

Bedside Body Mechanics

Caregiving activities often involve frail and disabled people in bed. Our backs are vulnerable to injury from prolonged leaning and bending when we provide bedside care. The good news is that the use of body mechanics can be tailored to bedside care! The following tips limit back strain when caregiving for people in bed:

- If the bed has side rails, lower the side rail on the side where you are working.

TABLE 9.1   Examples of Good Body Mechanics

1. Plan ahead and secure all the equipment.
2. Get close to the load.
3. Communicate with your lifting partner and the person being lifted.
4. Test the load before lifting.
5. Counterbalance the load by shifting your weight back to decrease strain.
6. Lower your center of gravity for the lift.
7. Bend knees and lift with legs.
8. Keep back vertical, maintaining the three natural curves.
9. Avoid overreaching with arms, keep shoulder blades pulled back.
10. Tighten abdominal muscles during lift.
11. Avoid twisting the back.
12. Pivot feet with body when turning.
13. Get a second person if you feel uncomfortable.
14. Do not complete the lift if it doesn't feel safe.
15. When working over the bed, put the rail down and kneel on the bed.

- Place one knee on the bed when helping a person roll or scoot in bed.
- Use a drawsheet under the person for leverage and comfort while moving in bed.
- If possible, adjust the bed height so that you are comfortable, and avoid leaning over.
- When rolling a person over, have the person assist by first bending his knees up then pulling on the side rail in the direction of the roll.
- When washing a person's back, position the person in bed lying face down, propped on pillows partway under the shoulder and hip. This position relieves you from holding the person with one hand while attempting to wash with the other.

Basic Safety Considerations

- *Plan ahead.* Think through the details of the transfer. Know what method to use and how many people are needed. Have all equipment needed close by. Know the person's physical and mental limitations and which side to go to.
- *Equipment (such as beds, wheelchairs, and shower chairs) needs to be in good working order.* This includes effective brakes, removable armrests, and adjustable height. Whenever possible, adjust the bed height so the transfer surfaces are equal, or make the second surface slightly lower to avoid transferring "uphill."

- *Stabilize equipment before a transfer.* Don't trust the "wheel brakes" on beds and shower chairs! Place them up against the wall or against something heavy to keep them from moving during the transfer.
- *Recognize situations that require the assistance of a second person.* If the person has poor trunk control and is unable to sit independently at the edge of the bed, a second helper is needed to get behind and to help with balance during the transfer. It is necessary for the helper to get up on the bed close to the person being lifted. The helper should assist under the person's buttocks, using a barrier such as a towel or Chux to protect both the person and himself. Gloves may be necessary when doing a shower transfer.
- *Use a transfer belt.* A regular belt with a buckle can also work. It prevents our instinct to grab hold and pull on the person's arms—which can hurt. Place the belt low on the person's hips at a 45-degree angle from seat bottom. This position is more comfortable for the person and provides a more effective line of pull around the person's center of gravity. Figures 9.7a, b, and c provide an example of transfer belt placement.
- *Always block the person's knee with your knees from the moment he is at the edge of the bed until he is all the way back on the chair.* This prevents the person from sliding forward off the surface and helps prevent buckling during the transfer. Position one of your knees IN FRONT of the person's knee, with your other knee along the side. Be careful not to squeeze the person's knee from both sides—instead, your knees provide support in the front and along the side of the person's knee (see Figure 9.3). It is recommended to block only one of the person's knees to control the transfer. If needed for comfort, a hand towel can be folded and placed against the knee for padding.
- *Never assist any person's transfer by pulling or holding on to his arms.* Serious injury to the shoulder joint of the person being lifted can occur, it is uncomfortable, and it gets in the way of the person's normal movement pattern. It also limits the person's ability to help.
- *Do not allow the person being transferred to hold on to your neck, shoulders, or arms.* This can cause serious injury to your neck and shoulders. If the person is unable to push up from the surface

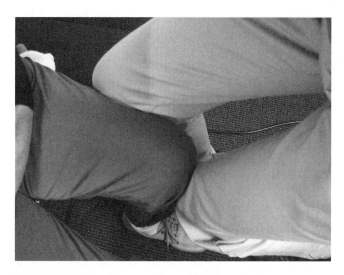

FIGURE 9.3   Correct knee block technique.

with his arms, as a last resort ask him to hold on to your waistband or belt. This often feels very secure to the person being transferred and is a safer option for you.

- *Do not undress the person during the transfer.* Do it before or after. The transfer is challenging enough without trying to manage clothing at the same time.
- *Be prepared for the unexpected.* There should always be a safe "way out" during the transfer if the person becomes unresponsive, combative, or frightened. The scoot method of transfer (described in the following section) allows the person to sit down even in the middle of a transfer, providing you with a chance to reposition for better body mechanics.

Communication Basics: Share Your Plans

A transfer can be a very traumatic experience for a person who is dependent. Many factors can heighten feelings of fear, anxiety, and pain. The person's perception of the transfer can be affected by mental impairment as well as by poor eyesight and hearing, poor balance, vertigo, pain, and personal issues. Anxiety and a heightened sense of vulnerability can be compounded during a bath transfer, when the person is undressed.

The thoughtful use of words and cues can improve the transfer experience for the person. Build trust by reassuring often, validating the person's feelings and concerns, and giving clear cues. Use the following strategies:

- *ALWAYS speak to the person at eye level.* Squat down because eye contact is important.
- *Be flexible.* Give the person some choice as to time or method.
- *Adjust for deficits.* Ask the person if he/she would like to wear glasses and hearing aids during transfers. Gestures work very well for persons who are hard of hearing or cognitively impaired. A dry erase board can be used with persons who are deaf or who cannot speak.
- *Explain.* Tell the person who you are and the goal of the transfer.
- *Appear as if you have all the time in the world.* Give the person ample time to react to your request and do not start moving the person until you see him initiating the movement.
- *Invite the person to help you.* Most people will do all they can to help. Say "I would like to help you . . ." instead of "I am going to . . . ." This implies that the person is actively involved in the activity rather than having some procedure "done to" him
- Use words that imply security, such as "hold on here" or "grab this for balance." Avoid words like "lean forward" and "move to the edge" that provoke anxiety in an anxious person. Instead, instruct the person to "put your head on my shoulder." Praise the person's efforts to help, no matter how small.
- *Smile.* Often.
- *Reassure the person that you will not let him fall.* Acknowledge that it may feel scary to move this way. Be sensitive about what is said in front of the person. For example, to avoid feelings of anxiety, don't say "I've never done this before" or "My back is killing me today."
- *Keep directions short and simple.* When two helpers are involved with a transfer, identify who will be directing the person to avoid confusion and distraction.
- *Stop the transfer.* Stop if the person becomes combative or terrified despite your reassurances.

Choosing an Appropriate Transfer Method

The Transfer Progression Continuum (Figure 9.4) provides a visual reference for different types of transfers. They range from independent to dependent. As a person's needs change for better or worse, the type of

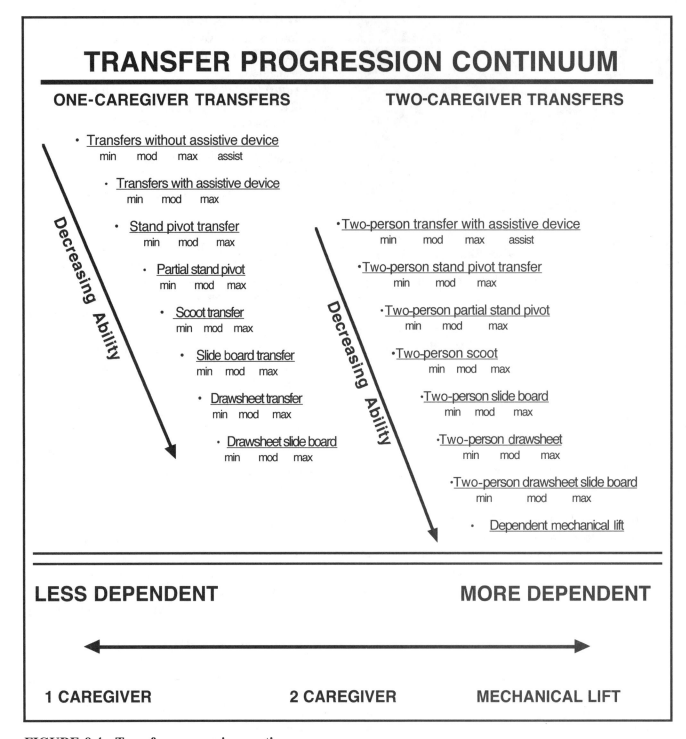

FIGURE 9.4 Transfer progression continuum.

transfer method should change. The goal is to maintain the highest level of function and safety.

The transfers identified down the continuum provide increasing caregiver assistance as the person's ability declines. The transfers are organized to identify choices depending upon the specific situation, the person's abilities, and the number of helpers required. For example, as a person with dementia experiences a decline, the transfer method will "slide down" the continuum. Alternatively, you may choose a two-person assist in recognition of physical difficulties, behavioral issues, or an awkward environment. We strongly recommend

TABLE 9.2 Choosing an Appropriate Transfer Method

The following questions are useful guides for choosing an appropriate transfer method.

1. *What is the person's sitting balance? How much assistance does this person need to sit upright?* Two caregivers may be needed to safely transfer a person with poor sitting balance.
2. *What is the length of time that a person can comfortably sit?* This assessment is important for pacing plans. A shorter sitting tolerance requires that the transfer be done with efficiency and advanced preparation.
3. *What is the person's ability to stand and bear weight through the legs?* Appropriate transfers for persons with poor weight-bearing abilities include the scoot, sliding board, or draw-sheet methods.
4. *What is the person's skin tolerance to sitting on different surfaces?* Assessing the skin's sensitivity is a first step in minimizing skin abrasions and tears. The second step is to adequately pad the surfaces of all equipment used in the transfer.
5. *What type of equipment is necessary for the transfer and bathing technique?* For example, will the person need a backrest or removable armrests or a bath blanket to pad the equipment (i.e., slideboard)?

---

that mechanical lifts be used only after two-caregiver transfers have been attempted.

The choice of transfer varies according to the amount of aid required by the person and the number of caregivers assisting with the transfer. The best transfer method for a given situation reflects the person's physical abilities as well as behavioral, environmental, and resource issues (Table 9.2). There needs to be a balance between assisting enough and not overassisting. Standard definitions have been developed and are widely used:

- minimal assistance = person can assist 75%, caregiver must assist 25%
- moderate assistance = person can assist 50%, caregiver must assist 50%
- maximum assistance = person can assist 25%, caregiver must assist 75%.

Assessing how much help the person needs allows you to maintain the person's functional abilities and prevent injuries to the person and to yourself.

An initial physical therapy or occupational therapy evaluation should be done to determine the person's strength, range of motion, and safest transfer method. However, recognizing that changes in people's strength and health occur, you should examine the person's transfer needs on an ongoing basis.

Preparing the Person for the Transfer

The first step in any transfer is to prepare the person by getting him into the "ready" position prior to every transfer.

- Have the person scoot forward to the edge of the seat to the point that he cannot see the chair or bed between his legs. This movement occurs by shifting weight onto one hip at a time. You can squat in front of the person and assist with one of your hands from behind the person's hips. Pull forward, alternating sides as needed.
- Place the person's feet back so the person's toes are directly under his knees.
- Ask the person to sit up straight and bend forward so that his shoulders are over his toes.
- Cue the person to push up from the surface (armrests) with both hands, if able.

Use a consistent cue so the person knows when he is to move. It is helpful to use three rocking motions and the verbal cues "one, two, three," with movement occurring on "three." This rocking phase can help relax people who are stiff and rigid and make leaning forward easier. You need to stay out of the person's way as he leans forward by lowering your center of gravity, squatting, and keeping your back straight.

Taking the time to prepare for the transfer eliminates unnecessary lifting. Although the person may not understand what you want him to do, scooting and leaning forward often trigger an instinct to stand. Cognitively impaired persons can better understand what they are supposed to be doing if you assist them into the "ready" position. This strategy also provides a weight-bearing opportunity through the arms and legs.

Specific Transfer Methods

The following methods are presented according to the person's abilities, progressing from fairly independent to more dependent.

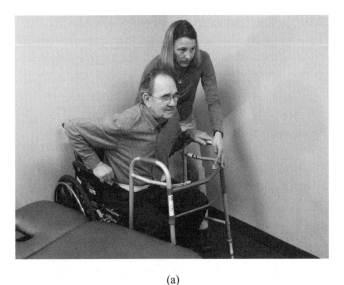

(a)

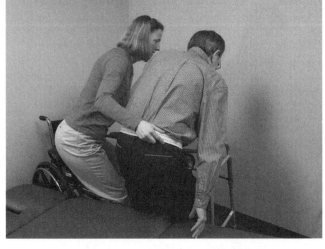

(b)

FIGURE 9.5 Walker transfer.

Walker Transfer

(Figures 9.5a and 9.5b)

Purpose: Assists a person with a walker to stand, turn, and sit down.

Skills: For people with fair balance and the ability to bear considerable weight through their arms and legs. Usually, one caregiver is required.

Procedure:

a. Prepare the person: Scoot him forward. Place the person's toes under his knees. Have the person lean forward, get his nose over his toes.
b. Place a transfer belt around the person's waist.
c. Position yourself beside and slightly behind the person. When a person with a walker loses balance, he almost always falls backward.
d. Have the person push up from the sitting surface with at least one arm. Do not pull up with the walker—it can tip over.
e. Once standing, place both hands on the walker for balance.
f. The person should then step around to the next sitting surface, holding on to the walker and backing up to this surface until the backs of both legs are touching the seat.
g. Have the person sit by bending forward at the hips, reaching back with both hands to touch the seat

(or armrests). Now ask the person to sit slowly bending knees in a controlled manner.

Stand Pivot Transfer

(Figures 9.6a and 9.6b)

Purpose: Assists a person to stand, turn without use of a walker, then sit.

Skills: For people who can bear weight while taking a few small steps.

Procedure:

a. Prepare the person: Scoot him forward. Place the person's toes under his knees. Have the person lean forward, get the person's shoulders over his toes.
b. Place the transfer belt around the person's waist.
c. Standing in front of the person, block the person's knee by placing your knees in front and alongside of his (Figure 9.3).
d. Holding on to the transfer belt, rock the person forward over his feet, counting "one, two, three" and moving on three. Each rock or count should lean the person farther forward until the person's shoulders are over his toes and he is ready for "lift-off." As the person leans forward, you should sit back and keep your back straight (as if you are sitting in a chair).

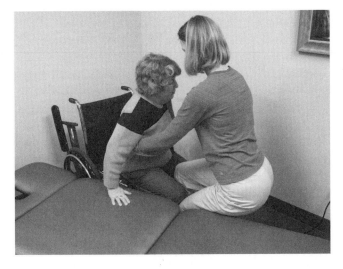 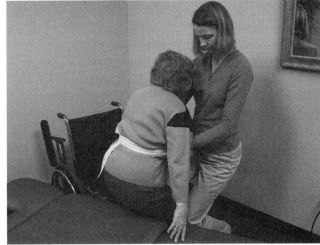

(a)   (b)

FIGURE 9.6   Stand pivot transfer.

e. On "three," help the person stand by supporting the person's hips with the belt and by supporting his knee with your knee block.

f. Once standing, it may help the person to hold onto an additional belt around *your* hips as the person steps around and back up to the second surface.

g. Have the person sit by bending forward at the hips, reaching back to the armrest or sitting surface, and slowly lowering to sit. Throughout the transfer, maintain support by using the belt on the person's hips and your knee block on the person's knee to prevent buckling.

Scoot Transfer

This method protects your back from twisting during a lift and allows you to complete the transfer in a number of small movements with opportunities to reposition yourself and the person. The movements are smaller and slower, which decreases the fear of falling and anxiety in the person being transferred. The scoot transfer requires little ability and prevents injury to the person's hips, knees, and ankles, which are vulnerable to twisting during the traditional stand pivot transfer.

Purpose: Helps a person move from one sitting area to another in a series of two to four small scoots as opposed to one standing or pivot movement. Ideal for transfers to bed, chair, commode, or shower chair.

Skills: The one-caregiver transfer is for people with good trunk control and balance in a sitting position. It can be performed as a two-caregiver transfer for those who need assistance to remain in a sitting position.

Procedure: One caregiver

a. Prepare the person: Scoot him forward. Place the person's toes under his knees. Have the person lean forward to get his shoulders over his toes. Remove armrests because small movements will occur and the person will not be lifted high enough to clear the armrest.

b. Place the transfer belt low on the person's hips at a 45-degree angle to the seat bottom (see Figure 9.7). Before the first scoot, determine the distance to be moved and tell the person how many scoots are anticipated.

c. Rock the person forward three times over his feet, with "lift-off" on three, clearing only the person's bottom and moving laterally just a few inches. Pull on the transfer belt to guide the person. A folded sheet or blanket can be placed to pad the surface and protect the skin.

d. Reposition your feet and the person's feet, and continue the process two or more times until the person is seated all the way back on the second surface.

Procedure: Two caregivers The first helper, positioned in front, gives cues to the person to avoid confusion. The

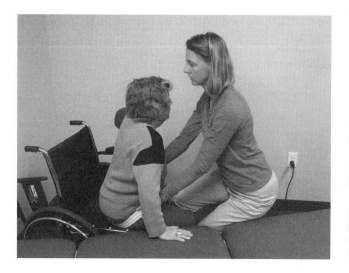

(a)

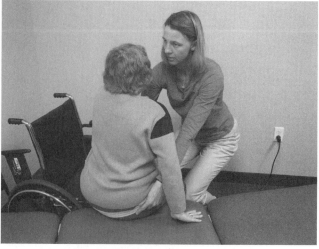

(b)

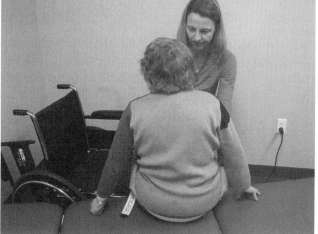

(c)

FIGURE 9.7   Scoot transfer—one-caregiver assist.

second helper assists from behind when the person has poor trunk control. It is the responsibility of the second helper to maintain the person's trunk position and to help the person lean forward.

a. Prepare the person: Scoot the person forward. Place the person's toes under his knees. Have the person lean forward, get his shoulders over his toes. Remove armrests because small movements will occur and the person will not be lifted high enough to clear the armrest.

b. The second helper gets behind the person in the wheelchair or up on the bed. The second helper assists the person in leaning forward with his shoul-

ders. The second helper then places hands under the person's hips, using a barrier as needed. This helps control the person's trunk by keeping the person's shoulders midline and over his feet.

c. The belt is placed as described earlier.

d. The front helper blocks the person's knee.

e. During the rocking phase, the back helper increases the person's forward lean with his shoulders. The back helper then places a hand under the person's hips to help keep the trunk midline while the front helper guides the scoot using the transfer belt.

f. The two helpers take turns repositioning themselves and the person after each scoot to maintain good body mechanics. The front helper maintains the knee block at all times.

Caregiver Wisdom

These transfers are a lot easier on my body. You can feel the difference. For example, usually the gait belt is placed around the waist for transfers. Here we place it on the hips and it is much easier for both the staff member and the person being moved. You get better leverage.

Deanna Peacock, CNA, Providence Benedictine Nursing Center, Mt. Angel, OR

Sliding Board Transfer

Purpose: Assists a more dependent person to slide from one sitting surface to another in a seated position, as with a scoot method. It is appropriate for transfers to bed, chair, commode, or shower chair when equipment has removable armrests.

Skills: This method is often used with persons who are more dependent. It uses a board approximately 10 inches wide by 20 inches long, strong enough to accommodate the person's weight. The slide board acts as a bridge between two different surfaces, providing firm support throughout the transfer process. Like the scoot transfer, this transfer can be performed with one or two caregivers. Sliding board transfers are optimally performed when a person is clothed or when a drawsheet is used. This transfer becomes difficult when a person is unclothed and wet, and additional precautions are needed when the technique is used with baths. See Table 9.3 for suggestions for protecting the skin during transfers.

Procedure: One caregiver

a. Prepare the person: Scoot the person forward. Place his toes under his knees. Have the person lean forward to get his shoulders over his toes. Remove armrests because small movements will occur and the person will not be lifted high enough to clear the armrest. Place the transfer belt low on the person's hips.

b. Sliding board placement: Ask the person to lean to the opposite side. Carefully lift the leg upward from the knee. Slide the board under the person at an angle toward the "sitting bones," or ischial

TABLE 9.3 Suggestions for Protecting Skin During Transfers

- Place a pillowcase or Chux over sliding board before placing it.
- Use talc powder to make the surface slick, absorb skin moisture, and reduce friction.
- An athletic supporter or "jockstrap" protects a man's genitals from being pinched while allowing the rectal area to be cleaned. A pillowcase can also be used to help hold the genitals up safely during the transfer (placed between person's legs like a brief) and can be carefully removed and replaced through the hole in the shower chair.

tuberosities. Look and ask while doing this to be sure nothing is getting pinched or poked by the board. The sliding board will form a diagonal "bridge" from under the person's thigh to the surface where he is moving (see Figure 9.8).

c. Block one of the person's knees with both of yours.

d. Rock the person forward three times to help him lean forward. On the count of three, "lift-off" and guide the person to scoot across the board.

e. Once the transfer is complete, remove the board by having the person lean away from the board. Lift the leg and gently remove the board

Procedure: Two caregivers

a. If needed, the second helper should assist from behind as described in the scoot method (see Figures 9.9a and b).

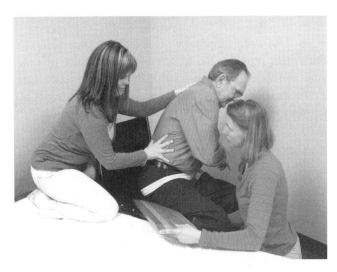

FIGURE 9.8   Sliding board placement—two-caregiver assist.

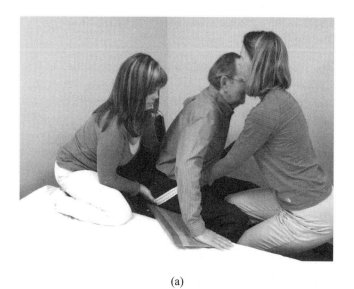

(a)

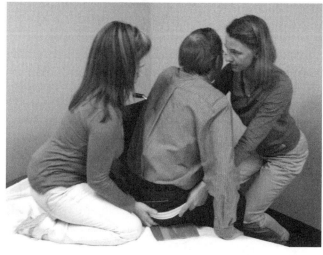

(b)

FIGURE 9.9   Sliding board transfer—two-caregiver assist.

b. The second helper stabilizes the board with one hand flat on the board, as the sliding board may move during the transfer (usually with the initial scoot).

Looped Drawsheet Transfer

Purpose: Assisting a person to transfer when wearing a transfer belt may be uncomfortable for the person or contraindicated by medical issues (such as abdominal incision, feeding tube, or colostomy bag). The method works well for a more dependent person needing to transfer to a commode and shower chair with removable armrests when the person is not clothed.

Skills: Use with persons who are more dependent. A drawsheet replaces the transfer belt as a point of control. The sheet increases comfort by dispersing pressure over a greater surface area. It can be done by one or two caregivers.

Procedure: One caregiver

a. Prepare the person: Scoot him forward. Place the person's toes under his knees. Have the person lean forward to get his shoulders over his toes. Remove armrests because small movements will occur and the person will not be lifted high enough to clear the armrest. Remember—this transfer does not use a transfer belt.

b. Bunch up a flat sheet, lengthwise, to form a long band 5–6 inches wide. Place this around the back of the pelvis of the seated person. Loop the sheet under the person's thighs in front, forming a "donut" for the person to sit on.

c. Block the person's knees.

d. Pull the sheet around the person so it is snug. One hand holds the sheet together on one side, even with the person's hip bones. The other hand holds on to "the donut" at the other hip. Leverage is provided via the snug sheet.

e. Rock the person forward and perform 2–3 or more small scoots, as described with the scoot and sliding board methods. Once the transfer is complete, the sheet is easily removed.

Procedure: Two caregivers

a. The second helper assists with this transfer just as in the scoot and sliding board transfers. The helper is again positioned behind the person, with hands under the person's hips. The second helper does not hold on to the sheet as this can cause it to slip (Figures 9.10a and b).

Making Therapeutic Transfers Routine Practice

A comprehensive transfer training program is the most effective strategy for providing therapeutic transfers and

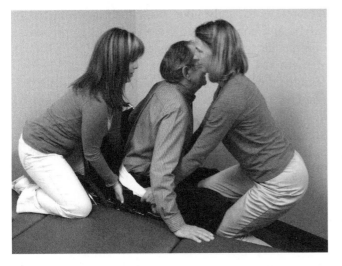 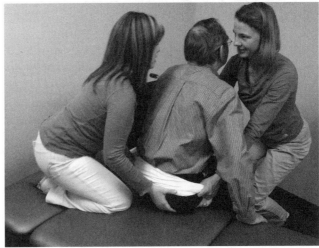

(a)   (b)

FIGURE 9.10 Looped drawsheet transfer—two-caregiver assist.

for minimizing the number and cost of caregiver injuries. This requires establishing policies, monitoring practices, and maintaining quality care and caregiver well-being. Suggestions for a transfer training protocol include:

- Make transfer classes MANDATORY for all who are connected with providing, supervising, or monitoring caregiving: CNAs, LPNs, RNs, medication technicians, supervisors, and resident care managers. Values, understandings, and expectations are more likely to be shared with an inclusive approach.
- Make classes long enough to provide instruction and hands-on practice of transfer techniques by caregivers under the instructor's supervision.
- Provide both basic and advanced classes. Advanced classes should include role-playing of case examples and group problem solving on difficult situations that arise with "real people." In this way, advanced classes become "case reviews" and "continuing education."
- Offer classes monthly, either as basic or as advanced classes. Provide a consistent class synopsis to participants and require that those standards be followed on the floor.
- Use a variety of interventions to sustain momentum, as described in Table 9.4.

TABLE 9.4 Strategies for Maintaining a Systemwide Transfer Program

Choose broad topics for inservice education programs.	• "PROMOTE FITNESS!" Inservice staff on back exercises for improved posture and strength. • "The pros/cons of mechanical lifts and when and how to use them." Establish and discuss guidelines for carefully assessing need. • "Communicating with cognitively impaired people." Invite a geriatric or mental health specialist.
Attend to the needs of the caregiver.	• Provide transfer belts for every person and *require* their use. • Survey the staff for feedback on effectiveness of transfer education.
Promote activities that involve unit-based teamwork.	• Schedule floor inservices for residents presenting transfer challenges, encouraging RNs to problem solve and assisting CNAs at bedside transfer sessions. • Provide detailed instruction on individual transfer method for staff via wall signs and bedside information sheets. • Videotape difficult transfers being done properly and leave on unit for staff to review together.
Evaluate transfer method choices as a quality assurance program.	• Use the transfer progression continuum to track the appropriateness of transfer methods for individual residents. • Track incidents involving moving residents and caregiver work-related injuries and intervene where needed. • Communicate tracking results to all involved.

Caregiver Wisdom

What I see happening in other places feels unsafe to me. It seems like throwing people into chairs with no warning. After learning these new techniques, I feel more in control. I use better body mechanics, being sure to stay low and use my legs more than my back. My back feels better.

Kim McCollum, CNA, Providence Benedictine
Nursing Center, Mt. Angel, OR

SUMMARY

A therapeutic transfer assists a person in a way that maintains and supports his/her abilities. This approach requires us to apply good body mechanics, attend to safety, and communicate clearly. The appropriateness of a specific transfer method depends upon the person's strength and balance. The transfer progression continuum identifies transfer methods that provide increasing amounts of assistance to address a person's increasing dependence. The success of a therapeutic transfer program depends upon the support of the facility's administration. We all benefit from practicing and promoting therapeutic techniques.

REFERENCE

Wood, J., Raudsepp, T., Miller, L., & Dazey, E. (2000). Improving resident transfers. *Nursing Homes: Long Term Care Management, 49*(2), 68, 70, 72.

CHAPTER 10

The Physical Environment of the Bathing Room

Margaret P. Calkins

Bathing typically happens in a room, which provides a visual, auditory, olfactory, thermal, and textural context. There are also spatial qualities of the room that can either cause problems, support independence, or support caregivers providing assistance. In general, space issues are the same regardless of the setting (home, assisted living, residential care, or nursing home), although some of the details may vary from setting to setting. Except when specifically noted, all suggestions in this chapter can be applied to all types of care settings. Suggestions will address both modification of existing bathing rooms and considerations for new construction. Since there is a separate chapter dealing with tub and shower equipment, this chapter concentrates on the environment around the tub or shower. Except as noted, the term "being bathed" refers to either taking a bath or a shower, and the term "bathing area" refers to a room or space where a bath or shower is given. Finally, the focus here is on rooms specifically designed for bathing and not on bedrooms or other rooms in which sponge baths or other forms of cleansing might take place.

Because the environment is experienced primarily through our senses, this chapter is organized by sensory modality. The greatest emphasis is always on how the person being bathed is experiencing the setting, with a secondary focus on the ways the environment can support the caregiver. To put yourself in their shoes, consider trying the exercise in Exhibit 10.1.

After you've been in the shoes of a person with dementia it will be easier to know what to change in the environment.

Visual Environment

Bathing areas in most long-term care settings are sterile, institutional, and frightening spaces filled with unfamiliar equipment—tubs with mechanical lifts or sides that open up and look like they might swallow you, chairs on wheels or gurneys with arms that look like construction cranes. There also may be soiled utility carts, scales, extra wheelchairs, and boxes of supplies through which the person must navigate. In homes, while there is likely to be less large equipment, the counters and ledges and other surfaces are often jammed with personal care products—three or four kinds of shampoo, conditioners, body soaps, several brushes and combs, a hair dryer, shoe-polishing kits, hair color kits—the list can go on and on. It's not surprising that the person who needs some assistance with bathing resists going into the room! One positive trend that is gaining in popularity in both nursing homes and assisted living settings is providing a tub or shower unit in the bathroom connected to the resident's bedroom. With only one, or sometimes two, people using this area, and with staff able to monitor the number of products stored in the room, these rooms are both tidy and familiar. Both rooms are helpful to individuals with dementia.

If you live or work with one of the first two options described earlier and find bathing challenging, there are a number of strategies that should be implemented. The first solution is to keep it simple.

Keeping it simple in shared residential settings includes:

- Moving unnecessary equipment out of the bathing area.
- Eliminating or hiding clutter—use more decorative containers to hold personal toiletries and make the cupboard they are stored in more decorative.
- Building partition wall or installing a pretty curtain to hide storage areas.

EXHIBIT 10.1   Bathing Exercise

Experience bathing from the care recipient's perspective:

- Put on sunglasses smeared with a little petroleum jelly.
- Have someone undress you in a bedroom down the hall, drape you in a sheet, and wheel you to the bathroom in a wheelchair or shower chair.
- Then have someone give you a bath.
- Think about the visual experience—what do you see when you enter the room, while you're in the tub or shower?
- How is the lighting? Is it in your eyes?
- What is the acoustic environment like—what are the most prominent sounds you hear?
- How does the room smell?
- Is the temperature of the room comfortable?
- Stand on the floor while you're still wet. How comfortable is that?

Keeping it simple in home settings includes:

- Storing items under the cabinet, not on the countertop.
- Limiting the number of shampoos, conditioners, and body soaps in the tub/shower area.
- Building an additional storage closet to hold toiletries and towels (Figure 10.1).
- Giving everyone a basket for holding personal care items, and if necessary, storing the basket in their bedroom.
- Covering mirrors—*only if they are causing a problem.*
    - Laminated print—could be attached with Velcro or magnetic strips.
    - Cover with wallpaper.

Once you've eliminated the visual clutter from extra equipment and supplies, the next step is to make the room more visually pleasing and supportive of independent functioning. This can be done in several different ways.

- Change the appearance of the room:
    - Add art visible when seated in the tub.
    - Add a shelf for holding decorative knick-knacks.
    - Put personal care items behind a closed or decorated door.
    - Paint the walls a bright, cheerful color (warm colors reflect back on the skin, making people look healthier, while greens and blues may make people look sallow).
    - Use patterned curtains, not plain color.

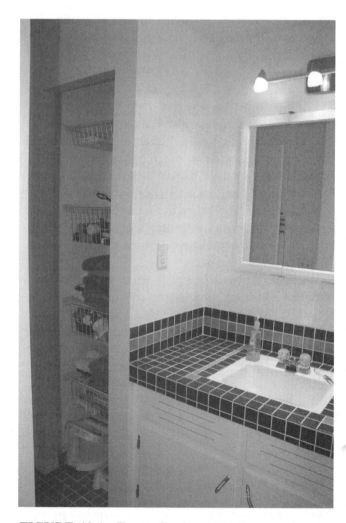

FIGURE 10.1   Example of good bathroom storage.

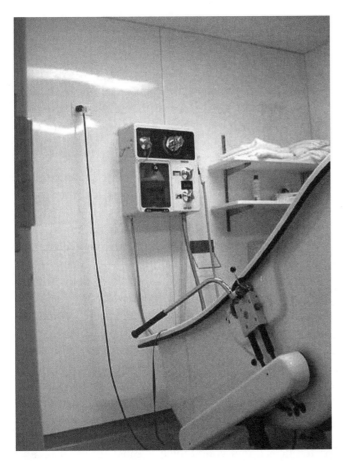

FIGURE 10.2   Undisguised control panel.

- Differentiated floor and walls of shower.
- Knickknacks that are brightly colored.
- Decrease visual contrast for items the person with dementia doesn't need to see. For example, sign or instructions for staff should blend into background surface.
- Support independence in people with dementia:
  - Laminate cue cards with steps of bathing process and mount in shower or hand to person using a tub.
  - Create an easily accessible location next to the tub/shower for these cards to be stored.

Finally, lighting is very important in bathing areas. It needs to be sufficient—particularly near the tub and shower—so you can see that the person is getting clean. If the person being bathed is looking up (in a reclined position or lying prone on a bath gurney), be sure no lights shine directly into his/her eyes. Get into the tub

- Disguise necessary "institutional" elements:
  - Relocate policy/procedure signage to be less visible.
  - Move the control panel for the tub or disguise it with a curtain (Figures 10.2 and 10.3).
- Add color and pattern to the room:
  - Decorative tiles—there are adhesive versions that can cover existing tiles.
  - Wallpaper border or stenciling at eye level for someone in the tub or shower. Water themes (beach, ocean, fish, penguins) are popular.
  - If there is a reclining tub, consider decorating the ceiling.
- Use visual contrast:
  - Increase the contrast of the edges you want the person with dementia to see:
    - Darker floor color to contrast with edges of the tub.
    - Tape along the top edge of residential tub to define.

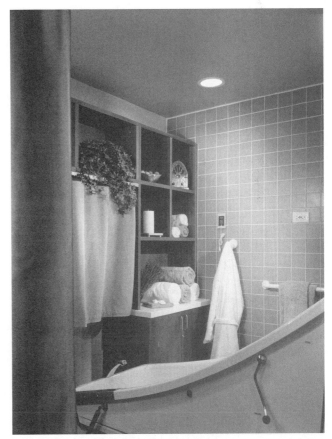

FIGURE 10.3   Disguised control panel.

or lie on the bath gurney and see what the person is looking at.

- Tips on lighting:
  - Sufficient so there are no dark shadows.
  - If people are lying down/leaning back (using tub chair or gurney) be sure they are not looking directly into lights.
  - Consider adding cove lights or wall sconces.
  - Install rheostat to adjust lighting levels for each individual.
  - Install several different types of lights that can be individually turned on or off.
  - Use full spectrum light bulbs—they help people look healthy, not sick (pale or sallow).

If all these principles are followed, then the bathroom will have a visually appealing look, it will not add to the distraction of the person being bathed, and it will support the caregiver(s) who are providing assistance.

Auditory Environment

Noise is distracting and can be agitating to persons being bathed. To reduce bathroom noise, there are two basic techniques. The first is to stop the noise at its source. Thus, the first and foremost rule is never bathe more than one person at a time—especially with people who do not particularly like bath time. Hearing sounds from another tub or shower and people talking (often speaking in a loud voice to be heard over the noise of the water or the whirlpool pumps) can be very distracting and disturbing. The second rule for stopping noise at the source is to keep the room private. Minimize intrusion from others when someone is being bathed. This is why it is so important to get extra soiled linen carts and stored equipment out of the bathroom when possible. The sound of someone opening the door and coming in is enough to elicit a negative response, fearing even more for the person's already compromised privacy.

The second basic technique is to keep noise reverberation down. Sound bounces off tile and other solid surfaces and floors. To reduce this reverberation and leaden noise use sound-absorbing materials. For example, add fabric-lined window and shower curtains. As a general rule of thumb, the fabric should be three to four times the width of the opening to have sufficient folds to maximize sound absorption. Another approach is to add water- and

mildew-resistant acoustic wall and ceiling panels. Wall tiles can be plain or decorative. The more walls and ceilings are covered by sound-absorbent tiles, the quieter the room.

Once negative noises and echoes are under control, you can consider the therapeutic benefits of adding positive sounds, such as music.

Methods for adding music:

- Create a library of new age sounds from nature as well as gospel, country, and classical music and show tunes.
- Install a radio/CD player in the bathroom.
- Identify each person's favorite, relaxing music and play it during bath time.
- Find music the caregiver and person being bathed can sing together ("I'm gonna wash that man right out of my hair" from "South Pacific" comes to mind as especially appropriate).

Most of these ideas will create an auditory environment that is more pleasant for caregivers and the person being bathed. Remember, however, that each person may have specific likes and dislikes. Classical music is soothing to some, just noise to others. Let the person's preferences direct your choice of music or other potentially positive sounds.

Caregiver Wisdom

I make sure the room is warm. If there's a heater in the room, I turn it up. If there is no heater, I let the water run before I bring the person in so it feels steamy and warm when we enter.

Mimi Leavenworth, Head CNA, Willametteview Convalescent Center, Portland, OR

Olfactory Environment

One doesn't generally think of the olfactory environment in relation to bathing, yet bathing areas are often characterized by lingering and sometimes powerful remnants of urine and excrement. Opening the door to a bathing area with these odors will certainly not get the bath off to a good start. The first tactic here is to attack at the source of the odor. Eliminate odors at their source.

Tips on eliminating odors:

- Minimize time soiled items (clothes, towels, trash) are kept in bathroom.
- Clean and disinfect hampers and floor where there have been accidents.
- Seal any cracks in seams (around toilet, at baseboards).

Once negative odors are minimized, you can consider adding positive aromas.

Methods for creating positive aromas:

- Use automatic room fresheners to keep room smelling clean.
- Use aromatherapy or essential oils; calming oils include marjoram, lavender, ylang-ylang, and clary sage.
- Use scented oils in the tub (check manufacturer's instructions if it is a whirlpool/hydrotherapy tub).
- Spray the room with air freshener.
- Use scented soap.
- Apply scented lotion or oil after the bath.

Remember, one size does not fit all. This is true of fragrances. Pay attention to personal preferences. Doing so will not only improve the olfactory environment, it may also help the person being bathed relax and enjoy the experience.

TACTILE ENVIRONMENT

Floors and Walls

As mentioned earlier, bathing areas are typically full of hard surfaces. This is important because of the moisture and the need to clean the area between baths. But hard, wet surfaces may be cold and do not make for a very comfortable experience. When you think of being comfortable, you typically think of being surrounded by warm, soft materials. Most people at home have either carpeting or a bath rug on the bathing area floor. Tiles are cold and uncomfortable on the feet—try standing around naked and wet on a tile floor and see how uncomfortable it is. While carpeting a bathing area in a long-term care facility may be impractical, having something soft on the floor can make a big difference to the experience.

Tips on increasing floor comfort:

- Use rubber-backed rugs (washable and nonslip).
- Install rubber flooring or look for flooring coating with a high coefficient of friction (above 80).

During the bath, a technique for improving the tactile environment is asking the person to hold a washcloth or sponge dipped in warm water. This may also encourage participation in bathing. If you are using a bath chair or bench, pad it or cover it with a towel to increase comfort.

You can also improve the tactile environment after the bath. Drape the individual in a warm towel. There is a range of commercial towel/blanket warmers available that are often used in facilities. At home use your dryer to warm towels. The person will enjoy this spa-like experience.

The issues are slightly different if the person is using a shower. Obviously the walls and floor of the shower must be hard surfaces, usually tile or other solid surface. Placing a rubber mat on the floor of the shower can make the surface soft and safe.

Grab Bars

It is critical to provide support for balance setting into the tub and in the shower, both when standing and when transitioning to a shower chair or bench. The location of grab bars in institutional settings is generally regulated by the Americans with Disabilities Act (ADA), although research suggests that these are not always the most useful locations for elderly individuals. The ADA regulations require a grab bar to the side of the toilet and behind the tank, mounted level to the floor, 33–36 inches above the floor. Many older adults find a side bar angled at approximately 45 degrees is better, because elderly individuals tend to pull themselves up rather than push down on a bar. There are also bars that can swing away or fold up, making it easier for a caregiver to provide assistance, should it be needed. In the tub or shower, there should be horizontal grab bars on all walls, 33–36 inches above the floor. Many institutional tubs come with grab bars preinstalled. While not required by the ADA, a 24-inch vertical bar at the point of entry into the shower/tub is also useful. All grab bars should be 1 1/2 inches in diameter and 1 1/2 inches from the wall. Other factors to consider when adding grab bars include:

- Use powder-coated rather than stainless steel, which is cold and institutional.

- Be sure grab bars contrast with the background color of the shower or tub.
- Purchase grab bars that are 24–30 inches.
- Install grab bars vertically at the front edge of the tub or shower to provide something stable to hold while entering.

Room Temperature

The temperature of the room is critically important to the comfort of the person being bathed. Older people are highly sensitive to drafts and are easily chilled. Anyone taking a shower is likely to have a significant amount of exposed, wet skin, which can quickly feel cold. Also, many of the tubs available on the market only cover the person being bathed from the waist down, leaving the upper portion of the body wet and exposed to drafts and chills. Thus, every bathroom should be equipped with an extra source of heat. If the caregiver is overly warm, almost to the point of sweating, the temperature is probably about right for the older person being bathed. Common sources of heat include heat lamps or radiant heat panels. Be sure the heat source is not a potential fire or electrocution hazard. No products that include exposed heating elements should be placed in a bathroom. Also, all heating elements should be mounted permanently to the wall or ceiling to avoid the possibility of coming in contact with water.

Finally, while not necessarily apparent to the person being bathed, it is extremely helpful to have at least one floor drain in all bathing areas. This helps deal efficiently with excess water should the shower or tub overflow. It also makes cleaning the room much easier. There are several excellent Web sites for home modifications for bathing areas. These are listed in the resource list at the end of this chapter.

Spatial Environment

There is much debate about whether bathing areas should be spacious (to provide room for caregivers and equipment) or cozy (to avoid that "institutional" feel). The answer, ideally, is both. And fortunately, these issues are not mutually exclusive.

Recognizing that many people need assistive devices (such as a wheelchair, walker, or lift), all bathing areas should provide sufficient space for use of these appli-

ances. The standard 5-foot turning radius specified by the ADA was not based on the needs of a physically frail older population with limited upper-body strength. Relatively few older individuals using wheelchairs can turn around in a 5-foot space with less than five or six turning points. A 7-foot radius is better. The ideal amount of space depends on the type of bathing equipment (shower vs. tub), other equipment (lifts, toilet, sink, vanity, etc.), and their location within the room. The best way to determine if there is enough room (particularly if you are considering new construction or major renovations) is to lay out the space and try it out. This process can be as simple as putting tape on the floor to designate the walls and fixtures or laying folding tables on their side to designate walls. Ask a typical user to try out the space to see how well it works. Be sure to include a caregiver in the space if the person being bathed needs assistance.

Ideas for creating user-friendly space:

- Bathrooms should have room to easily maneuver a wheelchair.
- Plan on a 7-foot radius specified so an older individual can easily maneuver independently.
- With new construction, build a mock-up of the room and have caregivers and residents try out the space to see how well it works before you build.
- Provide support for undressing and dressing in the bathroom.
  - Several hooks for hanging clothes.
  - Chair to sit on while dressing.
  - Small dressing table to do some grooming.

CONCLUSIONS

In long-term care settings, the bathing area is one of the strongest remnants of the old institutional model, where the goals of efficiency and utility still reign supreme over the psychological and emotional comfort of the person being bathed. But this can, and indeed must, change to reflect our changing cultural values about long-term care. If the priorities in long-term care are to recognize and support the cognitive, emotional, psychological, and spiritual needs of individuals as well as their physical needs, then all spaces need to reflect these goals. This is especially true for spaces where the most personal care—such as bathing—is provided. How a facility manages the minutia of life, such as the bathing process, including how bathing areas are designed and decorated, can speak volumes about the quality of a care setting.

At home, creating a pleasant bathing environment is also crucial. Keep the bathroom warm and free of clutter. Soften surfaces, reduce unpleasant noises and odors, and install grab bars. These simple changes can make bathing more comfortable for both you and the person you are bathing.

RESOURCES

Calkins, M. P. (2005). Designing bathing rooms that comfort. *Nursing Homes: Long Term Care Management, 54,* 54–56.

Kearney, D. (1992). *The new ADA: Compliance and costs.* Kingston, MA: Construction Publishers & Consultants.

Piner, T. (2003). Restoring dignity to bathing. *Nursing Homes: Long Term Care Management, 52,* 29–33.

Sabata, D. L. P., & Pynoos, J. (2005). Environmental coping strategies for caregivers: Designing and implementing online training for staff of family caregivers support programs. *Alzheimer's Care Quarterly 6*(4), 325–331.

Sloane, P., Honn, V., Dwyer, S., Wieselquist, J., Cain, C., & Meyers, S. (1995). Bathing the Alzheimer's patient in long-term care: Results and recommendations from three studies. *American Journal of Alzheimer's Disease, 10*(4), 3–12.

Warner, M. (1999). *Alzheimer's proofing your home.* West Lafayette, IN: Purdue University Press.

WEB RESOURCES

Rather than list specific manufacturers of products, which would be quickly out of date and far from comprehensive, this section gives readers guidance on how to look for more information on the Web.

Listserve for information on Alzheimer's Disease: alzheimer@wubios.wustl.edu

Web sites for general information on home modifications related to bathing areas (generally for the home): http://www.homemods.org/library/drhome/bathrooms. html (Accessed 6-14-07)
http://www.infinitec.org/live/homemodifications/ bathrooms.htm (Accessed 6-14-07)

Web sites for information on products used in bathrooms (these are both government-sponsored Web sites that are updated on a regular basis):
www.TechforLTC.org
www.ABLEData.com

List of useful search terms for other products:
Grab bars
Acoustic panels, moisture-resistant acoustic panels, acoustic panels for pools
Nonslip flooring, nonskid flooring, rubber flooring, high-friction flooring
Towel warmer (these tend to be exposed metal), blanket warmer (these tend to be safer cabinet style), warming drawer (less expensive than most hospital-grade blanket warmers)

CHAPTER 11

Equipment and Supplies

Stacey Biddle, Philip D. Sloane

Relaxing in a tub of warm water or under a gentle massaging spray from a shower are two of the simple pleasures in life. They tend to be overlooked when bathing a person with dementia. We often focus on maintaining cleanliness, removing bacteria, dirt, sweat, and debris from the body and improving one's appearance. The practical and pleasurable aspects of bathing depend on proper equipment, supplies, and education and/or supervision of a caregiver(s) in facilities or in the home setting. Bathing products are an essential part of the experience; they provide comfort and luxury as well as hygiene.

Bathing is often unpleasant for a person with Alzheimer's disease or a related dementia. A variety of caregiving strategies described throughout the book provide the cornerstone of effective bathing for persons with these diseases. However, equipment and supplies have an important role as well. For people with dementia, just as the general public, choosing the proper equipment and supplies can make the difference between a pleasurable, effective bath and an unpleasant, ineffective one.

This chapter discusses the wide range of bathing equipment and supplies available to caregivers of people with dementia. It focuses on shared residential settings (e.g., nursing homes and assisted living); however, much of the information is also relevant to family caregivers at home. Equipment related to showers, tub baths, and bed baths is described. Because individual products and brand names often change rapidly, the chapter concentrates on general principles and types of equipment rather than on specific products.

We would like to acknowledge Leanne E. Carnes as coauthor on the previous version of this chapter.

General Bathing Supplies

General bathing supplies are products that can be used in any bathing situation according to the needs of the person. Table 11.1 outlines commonly used bathing products.

Showers

Shower advantages:

- Faster, uses less water
- Allows for washing the body in sections.

Shower disadvantages:

- Less safe for those with balance problems or frequent falls
- Less effective in removing dried, crusted materials from skin.

Making the Shower Practical for the Person and Staff

Showering is the most common bathing method used by adults who live in the United States, including those who live in residential facilities. It is important to have easily accessible showers. Ideally, the person should be able to walk or be transitioned into the shower as easily as into a room, and caregiver access should be easy. There should be a smooth floor surface transition when entering the shower area. In combination shower-tubs like those found in many homes, where a smooth floor transition is not possible, the person must either be capable of stepping over the tub wall or must have another means of getting into the shower (see Bathtubs section). Also,

TABLE 11.1   General Bathing Supplies

General bathing supplies are products that may be used in any bathing situation, according to the individual needs of the person.

Product	Purpose	Description	Options
Liquid soap	Clean skin without overdrying	A liquid product that is applied to wet skin and then rinsed off to remove dirt and odor	Fragrance Nonlathering
Liquid lotion soap	Skin conditioning and cleansing in one	A liquid product that cleans and moisturizes the skin	Rinseable No-rinse
Bar soap	Clean the skin	Traditional method of cleaning the skin, needs water to apply and remove	Fragrance Moisturizer Texture
Incontinent cleanser/ deodorizer	Clean the perineum area between baths	Product that when applied cleans and disinfects; does not require water to rinse	Gel Foam Liquid Liquid spray Moisturizer
Body wash and shampoo	Clean entire body from head to toe	A combined product used to clean the body, face, and hair	Moisturized Fragrance Gel No-rinse
Shampoo	Clean hair	Traditional method of cleaning the hair; requires water to apply and remove	Fragrance Hair type Dandruff
Shampoo conditioner	Hair moisturizing and cleaning in one	A product that cleans and moisturizes the hair	Rinseable No-rinse Fragrance
Conditioner	Moisturize hair	Traditional method of moisturizing the hair	Rinseable No-rinse Fragrance
Dandruff shampoo	Clean hair and aid in the cessation of dandruff	A shampoo product; requires water to rinse	Prescription Nonprescription
Lotion	Moisturize skin	Traditional method to moisturize the skin	Fragrance Thickness
Washcloth	Aid in lathering/agitation of cleansing products; remove dead skin cells	A small cloth used for spreading and agitating cleansing products	Woven Nonwoven Colors
Towel	Dry the resident; keep resident warm	Large absorbent cloth	Woven Nonwoven Colors
Disposable washcloths	Decrease the spread of contaminants	One-time-use washcloths for cleaning	Prepackaged with cleanser Size
Examination gloves	Prevent disease transmission	Protective barrier between caregiver and resident	Latex Vinyl
Deodorant	prevent body odor	Product applied to underarms to prevent odors	Stick Roll-on Spray
Tooth swab	Oral cleaning scrubber	A soft tip on a stick to clean teeth	Foam tip Rubber tip Fiber tip

(continued)

TABLE 11.1   *(continued)*

Product	Purpose	Description	Options
Toothpaste	Clean teeth	Oral cleaner	Tartar control fluoride Gel/paste
Toothbrush	Lather/agitate oral cleaner	Oral cleaning utensil	Electric Manual
Shaving cream	Prevent cuts during shaving; moisturize face	Topical product applied to face for shaving	Gel Foam Cream
Toe washer	Wash between toes	A thin stick with a scrubber on the end	Foam tip Rubber tip Fiber tip
Incontinent commode bath	Wash perineum area between baths using soap and water without giving the person a full bath	A toilet seat attachment that rinses the soiled area	Adjustable water pressure
Perineum wash	Clean and disinfect perineum area; can be used during and between baths	Cleansing product for very soiled areas	Rinse No-rinse Gel Liquid foam Moisturizer
Disinfectant cleaner	Clean and disinfect the bathing area	Disinfectant-type cleaner used for infection control after every bath	Scrub-free liquid Foam

whenever possible, showers should use a shower curtain or a hinged door instead of a sliding door, because sliding doors always block half of the opening, thereby limiting access.

The shower area should foster easy bathing. Products for cleaning the person need to be close at hand, unless there is a risk of the person grabbing or misusing the products. Then the products should be placed in reach of the caregiver only. It is best if the handheld showerhead is in a position where the hose will not drag across the person. Towels and extra washcloths should be close at hand, making the bath as easy and as quick as possible.

The shower should be strategically placed within the bathing room. It should be beyond visual range from the door so that (a) the way out is not seen, and (b) privacy will not be lost if the door into the bathing area is accidentally opened.

There should be a place for the person to sit in the shower. Fatigue will be minimized in the seated position, allowing the person to assist in the bathing process when possible. This can be accomplished using a built-in seat, a removable shower chair, or a shower gurney (described later in this section); however, tub or in-room bed bathing alternatives are often preferred to a shower for persons who are unable to sit or stand safely.

Safety Issues in Showers

The safety issues vary according to the shower's layout and accessories. Floors in a shower are wet and can be slippery, so nonslip flooring is essential. If a shower chair is used, a twist, lean, or slip may cause it to topple. To avoid this, some chairs can be locked into the walls of the shower. Other chairs have wheels that lock and nonslip surfaces on the bottom of the chair.

Hot water burns may also occur in the shower. As people age, their ability to respond immediately to a sudden rise in water temperature is often slow or delayed, thus increasing the risk of burns. A first-degree burn can result from a 20-second exposure to water temperature of 130 degrees Fahrenheit (a common temperature in hot water heaters). Third-degree burns can occur with as little as 5–6 seconds of exposure to water between 135–140 degrees Fahrenheit in an elderly person. Antiscalding devices are, therefore, highly recommended to alleviate this problem. The various types include those that attach to the water heater or those that are built into or added onto the tubs and showers. They are designed to prevent water temperatures from getting too hot. The water in a water heater with an antiscalding device should be set to approximately 125 degrees

TABLE 11.2 Available Shower Style Products

Custom (or General) Residential Shower Stalls

- Typically found in personal residences.
- Usually consist of three plastic or tile walls, a door, and an elevated drain platform (floor slopes to a central drain).
- Have the option of adding or installing grab bars, seats, and a ramp.
- Door can be hinged or sliding, or replaced with a curtain.

Roll-in Showers

- Have a barrier-free entrance.
- A gradual ramp leads up to the entrance, and the shower base slopes down to a central drain.
- Most entrances are wide enough for wheelchair passage.
- Option of door or a shower curtain.

Seated Shower Cabinets

- Looks like a tub but are not meant to hold water.
- Come with a built-in seat, a handheld showerhead, and a door.
- Seat may slide in and out of the tub to help ease of transfer.

Shower-Tubs

- Combine a bathtub and a shower.
- Come with the option to install an attached or unattached bath seat, transfer bench, grab bars, and handheld showerhead.
- May have sliding door or shower curtain.

Fahrenheit and between 104–106 degrees for tubs and showers.

Many people prefer to stand in the shower because it is more familiar and it gives a sense of control. Others are asked to stand because that position is better for washing the genital and anal areas. To reduce falls among those who stand, grab bars need to be easy to find, reach, and grip by people of varying heights. Grab bars should be strategically positioned in locations where a person is likely to transfer or stand up from a chair.

Cleaning and Maintaining Shower Areas

When multiple people use the same shower, as in care facilities, the showers must be disinfected after every bath, but few come with disinfecting systems. The walls, floor, and grab bars are all parts of the shower that need to be cleaned. A grooved tile surface is more difficult and time consuming to disinfect than a smooth fiberglass surface.

The drain needs special attention. The drain must be cleared of all residue from the previous shower. A second drain catch can be placed under the first drain catch to prevent larger debris from going into the pipes. This will help prevent the pipes from being clogged and water from resurfacing inside the drain.

Available Shower Styles

There are a variety of shower styles available as outlined in Table 11.2. In determining the most suitable shower style, the accessibility, comfort, and safety concerns of all users of the shower should be factored into the selection of a product.

Shower and Bath Accessories

Shower and bath accessories are products that can be added or built into the shower or added to the bathtub. Shower and bath accessories are listed and described in Table 11.3.

Bathtubs

Tub bath advantages:

- Can be luxurious and relaxing
- Can loosen dried and crusted debris and skin
- Can soak wounds.

Tub bath disadvantages:

- Can be difficult for persons with physical disabilities to get in and out
- Caregiver access may be difficult, leading to increased risk for back injury
- May take more time than a shower or bed bath.

A tub bath is traditionally considered the most relaxing and luxurious method of bathing. Oils, bubbles, and other products have been developed for tub bathing that can add to this feeling of luxury. The tub bath also has the advantage of allowing the person to soak, thereby

TABLE 11.3   Shower/Bath Accessories

	Accessory	Description	Options	Comments
	Antiscald device[1]	Easy to install screw on device; turns off water if temperature gets too hot	Different models for sinks and showers	Activates at approximately 117 degrees F
	Handheld showerhead[2]	Mobile showerhead with pressure control	Pause and/or on/off controls on the head White or chrome Metal or plastic extension tube	Allows for more controlled rinsing. Easier access for hard to reach areas on body
	Attachable grab bar[2]	Removable grab bar that fastens on the side of the tub	Plastic or metal	An alternative to a permanently fixated grab bar
	Standard bath/shower bench[2]	Durable seated bench for placement in tub or shower	Adjustable height legs Holes in the seat for drainage Cut out handle openings on side of seat for hand placement	Lower cost option for people who do not require the additional support of a back rest
	Bath/shower bench with a back[2]	Durable seated bench with a back rest for placement in tub or shower	Plastic pipe or metal Variation in width Adjustable height legs	Allows for added back support and stability

TABLE 11.3 *Continued*

	Accessory	Description	Options	Comments
	Over the edge transfer bench[2]	Bench extends over the tub with greater seated surface area	Plastic or padded seat Adjustable height legs Drainage holes in seat	Promotes safety with transfers. A person's lower extremities can be assisted over the tub wall as an alternative transfer to stepping into the tub
	Rolling shower chair[3]	Portable chair for use in shower and can be used as a commode	Casters Commode Curve arm Footrest Drop arm Bucket Fabric colors Seat belt	Easier transport into shower area
	Shower gurney[3]	Transport shower gurney	Drop arm sides Reclining	Enables a person to shower while lying down

[1]Photo courtesy of Alzheimer's Store, 800-752-3238, www.alzstore.com
[2]Photo courtesy of Invacare, 800-333-6900, www.invacare.com
[3]Photo courtesy of Innovative Products Unlimited, 800-833-2826, www.ipu.com

loosening stubborn dirt and debris and relieving stiffness in muscles and joints. Finally, it is safer and more comfortable for people with mobility problems because the person receiving the bath does not have to support posture. Transfers can be hazardous, however, and must be done with care (see chapter 9, Transfer Techniques). The traditional bathtub is low and located in the corner of a room. This makes caregiver access difficult. When assistance is needed, however, a number of specialized tubs and tub products can make tub use easier.

Practical Issues

Getting into and out of the tub should be easy for the person. If the person has mobility or balance problems, tub entry and exit can be accomplished by means of caregiver assistance, a lift or door built into the tub, or by using a transfer bench or chair.

A lift, usually requiring one person to operate versus having two caregivers to assist in a manual transfer, increases the person's privacy. The lift also helps prevent caregiver injuries. On the downside, the lift also takes training and may be tedious to set up and operate. Also it can be a frightening experience for the person being bathed, especially if that person has dementia. Mechanical lifts are often noisy, and the noise and movement can be confusing or can feel threatening. Some facilities do not use tubs at all with residents who have dementia because, in their experience, lift use has caused distress. However, lift systems that do not raise the person high in the air can reduce this problem.

One nonlift transfer system is a door built into the tub. The door allows the person to walk into or be guided into the tub. The person then needs to sit in the tub while it fills, however, which can cause some persons to become cold and/or agitated. Newer tubs fill in less than 2 minutes, which is an advantage as long as the person receiving the bath does not become frightened by the sudden rush of water.

Transfer benches and chairs provide another no-lift solution. They allow for immediate submersion, and the tub can be filled prior to the bather getting into the tub. Transfer benches can help promote independence by allowing the person more control when entering the tub. They should generally be used with supervision, however, to decrease falls and frustration. For persons with severe mobility limitations or who resist care, the process of using a transfer bench can place strain on the caregiver's back. Use of proper back safety techniques is important.

Caregiver access is another important issue in tub selection. Some tubs are built high enough up so that caregivers do not need to bend. Others have a built-in motor that allows them to be raised and lowered. Others are built low and require caregivers to bend; in such situations caregivers can have the person sit in a chair or seat in the tub, or they can themselves sit on low chairs or stools to prevent back strain.

It is helpful if a tub allows easy access to every part of the person. Strategically placed grab bars enable the person to pull up or assist in pulling to one side and then the other so that the underside can be reached and cleaned. Mesh seats and seats with a hole(s) are available to increase access to the rectal and perineal areas. Some tubs provide jets or ultrasonic devices, which, while not directly providing caregiver access, can help loosen debris from these private areas. If the tub does not allow access to the rectal and perineal areas, another option is to wash those areas prior to or after the bath, perhaps with the person standing or in bed.

Safety Issues

Safety issues in tub bathing are many. One is the risk of staff injury from bending over or from transferring a person with impairment. Injury due to encountering hard or sharp surfaces, or due to accidental slips or falls, is an added risk. The risk can be minimized through proper equipment selection and training. Safety equipment includes ergonomically designed tubs, pressure controls on water outlets, antiscald temperature controls, prop-erly placed grab bars, a handheld showerhead with a pause or on/off control on the head, and nonslip surfaces.

Cleaning the Tub

A multiple-user tub must be disinfected after every bath; this is both a legal and a hygienic requirement. The disinfecting system can be a part of the tub or a completely different device(s). Some tubs (especially those with jet systems) come with a built-in disinfecting system; other bathtubs have to be manually disinfected. A recent study indicated that automatic disinfecting systems work well, but the study suggested that system bacterial counts may fluctuate more in tubs with jet systems; thus, facilities using jets need to be especially careful to clean the tub according to manufacturer instructions (Sloane et al., 2007). Most disinfecting systems have safety controls that prevent use in unauthorized times or when the system is malfunctioning. In either case the tub must be easy to clean. Easy to clean, nonporous surfaces are a common feature of most tubs.

Available Products

There are many products available when it comes to bathtubs and bathtub accessories. Because so many exist, and new ones appear frequently, this section will provide an overview of the basic types available. Table 11.4 describes the four major tub types: (a) residential tubs, (b) water agitation tubs, (c) tubs with a door, and (d) bathing tables. The first type is a general tub; the latter three types are specialized tubs, all of which have certain advantages.

Specialized tubs allow for different and sometimes very specific options for special populations. Among the features available in specialized tubs are entry doors, integrated lifts, bedside attachments, whirlpool jets, hydro sound, moveable/immovable seating, built-in grips and/or bars, and self-contained disinfecting systems. Not all people need specialized tubs, and no specialized tub is preferred by even as many as half of persons with dementia; instead, the different types of tubs each appeal to specific subgroups of disabled older persons. A person who has good physical function and relative independence can use the less expensive general tub (or a shower); persons who can sit upright and assist with transfer often do best with seated tubs (or, if they prefer, seated showers); and persons who are severely impaired often do best with recumbent tubs (or bed baths). Since

TABLE 11.4   Four Major Tub Types

Residential tubs

- Allow for atmosphere to be more similar to a private home.
- Can be adapted with the addition of grab bars and seats, nonslip surfaces, handheld showerheads, and antiscald temperature controls.
- Familiar to most persons
- Cost less than specialized tubs

Water agitation tubs (two types)

- Water agitation is used to massage skin, loosen stiff joints, and remove debris.
- Whirlpool systems have jets that circulate the water, often with pressure control features. Cleaning is more complex but in some tubs is done automatically.
- Hydro sound is water agitation without jets by the use of ultrasonic waves. Cleaning is simpler.
- Tubs vary in length and shape.
- Options can include: a door, an attached lift, a built-in seat, a removable seat, or no seat.

Tubs with a door

- Alleviate the need for a lift for persons who can assist with transfers.
- Allow the person to get in and out of the tub with little to no assistance.
- Door has a watertight seal, so the tub can fill without leaking.
- Water agitation systems and/or disinfecting and skin care systems are optional.
- Tubs vary in length and width.

Bathing table

- Mainly used for persons with severe disabilities.
- Table is an elevated flat surface with at least one drain and raised sides or railings.
- Mostly in bathing areas but can be assembled bedside if there is a place to drain the water.
- Allow the person to remain horizontal during the bath.
- Variety of surfaces—mesh cot, molded plastic, or nonporous fiberglass.

---

needs and wishes vary from person to person, it is impossible to find a single tub that works for all.

Bed Bathing

Bed bath advantages:

- Provides a gentle, private alternative for persons who fear tub baths and showers
- Requires less movement and transfer, thereby being especially suited for people who have pain during transfers
- Easier to do in segments, if a patient tires or becomes agitated quickly.

Bed bath disadvantages:

- Some people (mistakenly) feel that bed bathing doesn't get them as clean as a shower or tub bath
- Is usually not preferred by people who want independence in bathing.

Bathing a person in bed provides an effective and comfortable method of cleaning and hygiene for those who fear or dislike tubs and showers. It is valuable as an alternative for people who become upset or agitated during traditional baths. For those with severe mobility limitations it can also be a preferred bathing choice. No-rinse products (see Table 11.5) are available and can be an effective alternative to taking a bath or a shower.

Types of Bed Baths

There are three types of bed baths: the sponge bath, the bath in a bag, and the inflatable bed bathtub.

- Sponge bath is a bath given with a basin full of soapy water and a sponge or washcloth. After a body area is washed, it is rinsed with clean water with a sponge and then towel dried.
- A bag bath (two types) is a commercial product that can be purchased with the cleaning agents and towels already inside a microwaveable bag. In the other type, the towel bath, the caregiver mixes the cleaning agent and then moistens the towel or cloths (in-house packaging). The *covered massage bed bath*, a particularly gentle bed bath method, has been demonstrated to reduce agitation in some persons with Alzheimer's disease (Sloane et al., 2004). Downloadable directions for performing the covered massage bed bath and video training modules on preparing and

TABLE 11.5   No-Rinse Bath Accessories

	Accessory	Description	Options	Comments
	No-rinse products: shampoos, body wash, hand sanitizers.[1]	No water needed for application of most products.	Some products are concentrated and can be mixed with water for cost effectiveness.	Consider alcohol free to avoid drying of skin. Nonirritating formulas can minimize adverse skin reaction.
	Disposable washcloths in plastic dispenser.[1]	Premoistened washcloths in reclosable plastic bin.	Varied sizes and quantities.	Consider hypoallergenic.
	Soft pouch disposable washcloths.[1]	Premoistened washcloths in smaller quantity soft packs.	Can be used at room temperature or warmed.	Eliminates need for basins, soaps, linens, and lotions.

[1]Photo courtesy of Alzheimer's Store, 800-752-3238, www.alzstore.com

performing the towel bath are available at http://www.bathingwithoutabattle.unc.edu/

• Inflatable tub is a full-length bathtub made for bathing people in their bed.

Bed Bath Accessories

Most bed bath accessories are general products. A few specialized bed bath accessories exist. These include an inflatable bathtub, inflatable hair washing basin, head cradle, and bath blanket/sheets. The inflatable bathtub is designed to facilitate a bath in the bed. The hair washing basin is typically inflated and slid under the person's head while lying in bed; a notch on one of the sides cradles the person's neck. It drains by way of a tube in the base. The head cradle is similar to the hair washing basin, but the water is channeled off to the side for draining. And finally, bath blankets and sheets are useful for keeping bathers warm, comfortable, and dry. Blankets and sheets differ from each other in thickness and weight.

SUMMARY

Caregivers should take into consideration their current limitations in bathing a person with dementia in addition to the specific areas for improvement in the bathing processes. Bathing product information can be found on these free, government-sponsored Web sites: www.techforltc.org and www.abledata.com. Proper bathing of persons with mental or physical limitations requires considerable knowledge and skill. A wide variety of supplies and equipment is now available. If carefully selected and appropriately used, bathing experiences for both the person and caregiver can be significantly enhanced.

REFERENCES

Sloane, P. D., Cohen, L. W., Williams, C. S., Munn, J., Zimmerman, S., Preisser, J. S., et al. (2007). Effect of specialized bathing systems on resident cleanliness and water quality in nursing homes: A randomized controlled trial. *Journal of Water and Health, 5*(2), 283–294.

Sloane, P. D., Hoeffer, B., Mitchell, C. M., McKenzie, D., Barrick, A. L., Rader, J., et al. (2004). Effect of person-centered showering and the towel bath on bathing-associated aggression, agitation and discomfort in patients with dementia: A randomized clinical trial. *Journal of the American Geriatrics Society, 52*(11), 1795–1804.

RESOURCES

Brawley, E. C. (1997). *Designing for Alzheimer's disease: Strategies for creating better care environments* (pp. 45, 97, 196–202). New York: Wiley.

Day, K., Carreon, D., & Stump, C. (2000). The therapeutic design of environments for people with dementia: A review of the empirical research. *The Gerontologist, 40*(4), 397–416.

Mann, W. C., Hurren, D., Tomita, M., & Charvat, B. (1996). Use of assistive devices for bathing by elderly who are not institutionalized. *The Occupational Therapy Journal of Research, 16*(4), 261–284.

Sloane, P. D., Honn, V. J., Dwyer, S. A. R., Wieselquist, J., Cain, C., & Myers, S. (1995). Bathing the Alzheimer's patient in long term care: Results and recommendations from three studies. *The American Journal of Alzheimer's Disease, July/August*, 3–10.

Sloane, P. D., Rader, J., Barrick, A., Hoeffer, B., Dwyer, S., McKenzie, D., et al. (1995). Bathing persons with dementia. *The Gerontologist, 33*(5), 672–678.

Teresi, J. A., Holmes, D., & Ory, M. G. (2000). Commentary: The therapeutic design of environments for people with dementia: Further reflections and recent findings from the National Institute on Aging collaborative studies of dementia special care units. *The Gerontologist, 40*(4), 417–421.

Warner, M. L. (2000). *The complete guide to Alzheimer's proofing your home* (pp. 24, 165–171, 321–331, 387–399). West Lafayette, IN: Purdue University Press.

PART III

Supporting Caregiving Activities

CHAPTER 12

Bathing as a Vehicle for Change

Joanne Rader, Ann Louise Barrick, Darlene McKenzie, Beverly Hoeffer

INTRODUCTION

Imagine you are living in a care facility. It is 6:30 a.m. and you've just been awakened by a stranger, a caregiver, who says it's time for your shower. You don't want to get up, and you certainly aren't ready to be cold and wet. You politely refuse, saying, "No thanks. I don't like showers." The caregiver feels compelled to bathe you. You're on the schedule for today. She apologizes but says she has to get you up and bathed. She takes the covers off and insists you get up and hustles you off to the cold shower room. When you made the move to the nursing home, you didn't expect you'd be giving up your right to make choices about your daily life or refuse care that you didn't want! Yet, that is your experience, and the experience of many persons, with and without dementia. If you were at home you would have much more to say about how your care is provided. In a traditional care setting, like that just described, residents and caregivers alike too often have little to say about the circumstances of care provision. Shifting decision making to the bedside, to the caregiver and the resident, requires a "cultural" change at the organizational level. In this chapter we share strategies for transforming the organization so that decision making moves to the bedside. Many of these approaches have relevance for home and community-based settings as well. Finally, they apply to persons with and without cognitive impairment and their caregivers.

CREATING VALUE-BASED PRACTICES IN INSTITUTIONAL SETTINGS

Traditionally, the organizational structure of care facilities has been hierarchical, segmented into departments, with top-down decision making, with a focus on completion of tasks. The corporation or facility administration decides how care is organized and to a certain extent the general plan for how it should be implemented. Under this type of structure the nurse is responsible for seeing that the plan is implemented by the direct caregivers "under" her supervision. People who are frail and who have limited capacity to adapt are forced to comply with the pre-existing, regimented schedules and processes of the institution. They have to get up, eat, and go to bed on a time frame set up by the facility's organizational structure. It is common for someone to be denied a piece of cake or bacon if a staff member or the physician determines it is not good for them. Yet if the same person lived outside the institution, he/she would retain control of such decisions. Why shouldn't he/she have the same rights if he/she happens to live in an institution? A facility that espouses the values of dignity and choice but continues to force traditional bathing methods on fearful, reluctant residents, with no attempt to create a more flexible, pleasant experience, is not putting these values into practice.

Bathing can serve as a catalyst for improving care in general. Facilities are increasingly being put in the position of having to rethink the basic organization of care to meet the changing demands of the marketplace and of consumers, so re-evaluating your bathing methods and philosophy can inform this process.

Fortunately, since the 1990s there has been a growing movement to create more value-driven, person-directed care in facilities such as assisted living and nursing homes. Consumers, advocates, regulators, and providers realize that change is needed. Baby boomers, watching their parents, recognize that they are next, and they want something different for both themselves and their parents.

Many administrators and caregivers are actively working to create facilities where residents' needs and

TABLE 12.1   Paradigm Change From Traditional to Transformed Care Home

Traditional/Institutional	Transformed/Person-Directed
Medical/industrial	Social/holistic
Providing "treatments"	Nurturing the spirit
Task focus	Care matches needs, preferences
Rotating staff assignments	Consistent assignments
Administration/Staff make decisions about care	Residents make decisions about their care
All activities structured	Environment rich in opportunities for spontaneous activities in addition to structured
Schedule for convenience of staff/administration	Schedule adjusted for resident and staff needs
Facility "belongs" to staff	Facility is residents' home
Sense of isolation and loneliness	Sense of belonging and community
Departmental focus	Team approach with decision making at bedside
Budget decisions by administration	Decentralized budgets

preferences, rather than routine tasks and safety at all cost, determine how care is provided. For example, the time that people get up, go to bed, eat, and bathe are adjusted to the individual's wants and needs. Care recipients retain the right to have their choices respected and to take risks.

This important shift in philosophy of care is often referred to as culture change and requires re-examination of organizational and staff values as well as existing job descriptions, policies, and procedures. A result of this new paradigm is a transformation so significant that the values of the organization shift, driving a change in what's expected of all staff and often a different type of leadership and organizational structure (Baker, 2007; Fox, 2007; Shields & Norton, 2006; Thomas, 2004). The way care is organized, planned, and carried out changes dramatically (see Table 12.1).

Several individuals and organizations have emerged to champion this change and to shift away from what is "wrong" with nursing homes to create home wherever elders live. Four excellent examples are the Pioneer Network, the Eden Alternative, the Live Oak Institute, and the Household model.

Pioneer Network

The Pioneer Network is an umbrella organization for culture change founded in 1997. Its vision is a culture of aging that is life-affirming, satisfying, humane, and meaningful. It supports elders living in open, diverse, caring communities. The network works to create deep system change using the Pioneer values as the foundation (see Exhibit 12.1 for the list of Pioneer values). The Pioneer Network also works with regulators, advocates,

educators, researchers, consumers, and others to create systems that support choice and dignity for elders. (www.PioneerNetwork.net)

Eden Alternative and the Green House Model of Care

In 1991, Dr. William Thomas, a Harvard-educated physician, and his wife, Judy, created the Eden Alternative in a small nursing home in New York State. This

EXHIBIT 12.1   Core Values of the Pioneer Network

- Know each person and appreciate his/her uniqueness.
- Each person can and does make a difference.
- Relationship is the fundamental building block of a transformed culture.
- Respond to spirit, as well as to mind and body.
- Risk taking is a normal part of life.
- Put person before task.
- All elders are entitled to self-determination wherever they live.
- Community is the antidote to institutionalization.
- Do unto others as you would have them do unto you.
- Promote the growth and development of all.
- Shape and use the potential of the environment in all its aspects: physical, organizational, and psychosocial/spiritual.
- Practice self-examination, searching for new creativity and opportunities for doing better.
- Recognize that culture change and transformation are not destinations but a journey, always a work in progress.

Courtesy of the Pioneer Network © 2001, Rochester, NY

model focuses on addressing the three plagues of nursing homes identified by Dr. Thomas:

- loneliness
- helplessness
- boredom.

The core concept of the Eden Alternative is that facilities are for human beings, not places for the frail and elderly. The Eden Alternative supports homes becoming more person-directed through education and networking. It provides books, conferences, newsletters, videos, consultants, and support networks. More than 15,000 people have been trained as Eden associates and work toward meaningful culture change. This includes an emphasis on companionship and trust, encouraging staff and resident empowerment, decentralizing decision making, and enriching the physical and social environment through the introduction of plants, animals, and children as part of daily life. Over 300 nursing homes in the United States and around the world are registered as Eden Homes (www.edenalt.org). Registered homes commit to putting the 10 principles of the Eden Alternative into practice (see Exhibit 12.2).

Dr. Thomas went on to develop the Green House approach to long-term care. In this model, elders requiring skilled nursing care live in a cluster of freestanding small homes that each serve 6–10 people and that share resources and support services. Care is determined by personal choice and comfort and given in the context of a relationship. These intentional communities, led by self-directed household teams, were first built in 2003 in Tupelo, Mississippi. Currently there are plans to replicate the model in 50 projects across the United States. (www.thegreenhouseproject.com)

Live Oak Institute

The Live Oak Institute is another organization working for change. Since 1977 the founders, Barry and Debby Barkan, have created settings that provide care based on a deep respect for elders and the people who work with them. A hallmark of their work is the daily community meeting where elders, family, and staff come together to build connectedness and a place to learn, play, and grow together. Anniversaries, births, weddings, and deaths are celebrated and mourned together in the meeting, building a sense of belonging and family. (www.LiveOakInstitute.org)

EXHIBIT 12.2 The Ten Principles

1. The three plagues of loneliness, helplessness, and boredom account for the bulk of suffering among our elders.
2. An elder-centered community commits to creating a human habitat where life revolves around close and continuing contact with plants, animals, and children. It is these relationships that provide the young and old alike with a pathway to a life worth living.
3. Loving companionship is the antidote to loneliness. Elders deserve easy access to human and animal companionship.
4. An elder-centered community creates opportunity to give as well as receive care. This is the antidote to helplessness.
5. An elder-centered community imbues daily life with variety and spontaneity by creating an environment in which unexpected and unpredictable interactions and happenings can take place. This is the antidote to boredom.
6. Meaningless activity corrodes the human spirit. The opportunity to do things that we find meaningful is essential to human health.
7. Medical treatment should be the servant of genuine human caring, never its master.
8. An elder-centered community honors its elders by de-emphasizing top-down bureaucratic authority, seeking instead to place the maximum possible decision-making authority into the hands of the elders or into the hands of those closest to them.
9. Creating an elder-centered community is a never-ending process. Human growth must never be separated from human life.
10. Wise leadership is the lifeblood of any struggle against the three plagues. For it, there can be no substitute.

Courtesy of Eden Alternatives, 2007

Household Model

Steve Shields, LaVrene Norton, and others have created a framework for change known as the Household Model. By their description it is "not for people who seek a gradualist approach to change. It is for those who want revolutionary transformation in the culture of nursing homes and other long-term care settings." They provide a change matrix to guide facilities from the traditional model to the household model, looking at personal and leadership transformation, as well as at organizational and environmental change. In addition, they have created a toolkit, "Household Matters," that contains educational videos, downloadable policies and procedures and job descriptions, quality assurance programs, and a workbook for creating self-directed teams. All are designed to support facilities committed to replacing the institutional culture with "personal relationships; where small groups of elders—supported by self-led teams of employees—determine their own lives and build community" (Shields, Norton, Bump, & Maben, 2006).

These are just a few examples of how organizations and facilities are embracing care models based on such values as a deep respect for elders and an understanding of their right to live full and meaningful lives, with a voice in decisions made about their care. This is a big shift from the previous model based on safety at all costs and care focused primarily on the physical problems of elders. The new emphasis is on person-directed care and the promotion of health and wholeness.

Part of a transformed culture is for administrative and corporate personnel to understand that the way staff treat residents is a product of the way they are treated by management (Fox, 2007). Therefore, for elders to feel respected, supported, and seen, employees need to feel respected, supported, and seen. This is not only beneficial for residents and staff, it is good business. In our experience, facilities moving toward person-directed care and nurturing relationships between employees and residents reported greater ease recruiting and retaining skilled caregivers. Thus, if the organizational system is not designed with these goals in mind, a lot of money and effort will be spent on recruiting, training, orienting, and retraining caregivers entering and exiting through a revolving door. It has been estimated that the cost of turnover is about $2,500 per employee in direct and indirect costs (Seavey, 2004).

Specific care practices like bathing do not exist in a vacuum. They reflect the larger organizational culture. If a facility is committed to person-directed care, then changing bathing is an excellent practice to focus on first. The process will help identify organizational issues that need to be addressed to make culture change sustainable. The cost for changing bathing practices is minimal and primarily related to training. Most of what is required is support from administration and an attitudinal change for all staff.

Bathing can serve as a catalyst for improving care in general. Facilities are increasingly being put in the position of having to rethink the basic organization of care to meet the changing demands of the marketplace and consumers, so re-evaluating your bathing methods and philosophy can inform this process. The remainder of this chapter will illustrate some of the most important aspects of working toward institutional change in

New Organizational Emphasis

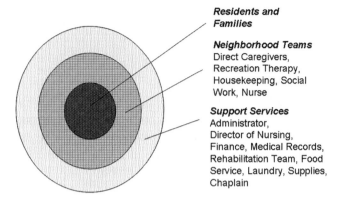

Residents and Families

Neighborhood Teams
Direct Caregivers, Recreation Therapy, Housekeeping, Social Work, Nurse

Support Services
Administrator, Director of Nursing, Finance, Medical Records, Rehabilitation Team, Food Service, Laundry, Supplies, Chaplain

FIGURE 12.1   At the center of good care.

the context of implementing person-directed practices in bathing.

TRANSFORMING BATHING CARE: KEY CONCEPTS

Moving Bathing Decision Making to the Bedside

A transformation to person-directed care requires decentralizing decision making, giving the resident and those providing care to the resident more authority. Figure 12.1 illustrates this new approach by placing the residents and families in the center circle. Direct caregivers, nurses, and other members of the neighborhood team who see residents on a daily basis are in the next concentric circle. Administration and other departments, located in the outer circle, are in service to those in the middle, encouraging and supporting decision making at the bedside.

This transformation to person-directed care is often a long and complex process. There needs to be support and a team focus that creates a more relational approach between caregivers and residents as well as a more consultive relationship between the nurses and the direct caregivers. Attitudes of flexibility and creativity are embraced. Roles change.

The Decision-Making Role of the Resident

In a transformed culture, the resident retains the right to refuse care or to make choices about how care is provided. This decision-making power and choice will help maintain the resident's highest possible level of independence and function. Caregivers are responsible for figuring out how to present and provide care that the resident agrees to and enjoys. If the resident has dementia, caregivers walk a tightrope, respecting the person's autonomy and independence yet making sure she receives assistance with decisions and the care she needs. If caregivers know their residents well, they will usually find, within the resident's past and current behaviors, solutions that respect preferences.

The Decision-Making Role of the Direct Caregiver

Direct caregivers need the authority and flexibility to make decisions about when and how residents are bathed for person-directed care to work. They are accountable and responsible for care. For example, if a resident refuses a bath or shower, they will try a variety of strategies to get the person to agree (getting him/her to "yes"). If the person still refuses, then the caregiver can determine what must be cleaned for compelling health reasons and has the skills to identify and carry out the most pleasant, least invasive way to do it. If the decision is to postpone the bath, then an alternative plan needs to be developed. If the person continues to refuse, then the caregiver can talk with her supervisor to find a solution to meet the needs of the person. It is not enough for the caregiver to simply say, "I asked her and she said no. It's her choice. There is nothing I can do."

Caregivers have frequently reported to the authors that if they try to adapt, postpone, or shorten bathing, they feel judged by their peers and supervisors. In the traditional culture, attempts to individualize the bath are sometimes seen as trying to "get out of work." This attitude needs to change. If the caregiver's job is viewed strictly as a series of tasks to be completed on a group of bodies (washing, dressing, feeding, toileting) day after day, and the caregiver is told what to do and how to do it, there is little reward and caregiving becomes an unattractive field of work. If instead the caregiver's job is viewed and supported as an opportunity to enter into meaningful and caring relationships, and the caregiver's input and opinions are important in care decisions, it provides a way for caregivers to be of service to others, and the job can become quite attractive.

The direct caregiver has unique knowledge, access, and responsibility for care. However, too often this knowledge has been ignored or not sought in the care planning process. For example, direct caregivers are often excluded from attending care planning conferences. In addition, unless their input is sought and used, caregivers may feel attendance is a waste of their time. Often, the usual staff members attending the conference (social workers, activities directors, nurse managers) don't have the same daily, direct access to the residents or the same knowledge of the person's care needs and preferences. Families and residents are now included in care planning as a result of the Omnibus Budget Reconciliation Act of 1987. The same needs to be done for direct caregivers.

The Important, Changing Role of the Nurse

Nurses have knowledge, training, and skills to assess complex medical situations that occur with frail elders. Many have additional skills for dealing with complex psychosocial issues. However, much of the nurse's time in traditional settings is tied up doing assessments, care planning, and documentation. Very little time is spent at the bedside. The old relationship model between the nurse and the direct caregiver is reflected in the commonly used title "nursing assistant." This seems to imply that caregivers are there to help the nurse complete her job, which has been defined as providing and overseeing the care of a group of people. The role and responsibilities in this dynamic are changing, with the licensed nurse becoming a supportive supervisor, there to assist the direct caregiver with problem solving and to model good care rather than to tell the caregiver what to do and to discourage (overtly and covertly) empathy and relationship.

Despite this shift, many nurses are still supervising in the old model where they "know best." Thus there can be a discrepancy between the degree of support nurses feel they provide to direct caregivers and the amount of support caregivers feel they receive. Direct caregivers sometimes view nurses as critical of their work and lacking understanding about residents' needs and wishes. For example, one nursing assistant reported to the nurse that she had tried various approaches with a person to get her to agree to a shower. From her knowledge of the person, she knew a shower that day would result in a battle. She shared this information with the nurse, who

EXHIBIT 12.3 Supportive Supervision

Supportive Supervision

- Provides education, modeling, and verbal encouragement
- Solicits and respects the knowledge of direct caregivers
- Supports flexibility and choice in the delivery of care
- Assures supplies and equipment are available
- Provides ongoing consultation and problem-solving assistance
- Provides "management by walking around" talking with residents, families, caregivers
- Holds caregivers accountable for bathing decisions
- Provides constructive feedback in a private setting when needed

---

Case Study

Moving to Person-Directed Bathing: Use a "Bathing Expert"

In a facility in Oregon, a very skilled CNA was asked by her supervisor to begin teaching her colleagues on the dementia unit about bathing. She worked with other caregivers to create person-directed bathing approaches for all residents living on the unit. This change greatly reduced the agitation and distress experienced during bathing. Considered the "bathing expert," the CNA, with the supervising nurse's encouragement and director of nursing's support, then went to other households that had challenging bathing situations and assisted at the bedside. Her expertise spread and new experts emerged.

---

told her to shower her anyway. The person was showered and the situation became a battle, ending with both nursing assistant and resident exhausted and distressed. On seeing them exit the shower, the nurse said to the resident, "There! Don't you feel better now that you are clean?" She was unaware of the huge cost in energy, esteem, and relationship that the shower had exacted from both parties.

In the transformed culture the nurse is part of a team that consults and supports, rather than simply directs (see Exhibit 12.3, Supportive Supervision). A supportive leadership model can work. For example, initially the purchasing supervisor in a facility in Oregon resisted buying the no-rinse soap product the nursing assistants (CNAs) recommended and ordered another product. The supervising nurse worked with administration until the no-rinse product the CNAs had requested was ordered. That soap is now a standard product in the facility. The nurse also worked with the laundry to create time-saving tools for the CNAs. At her suggestion, the laundry prepackaged the large towels and washcloths needed for the covered massage baths and placed them in the household linen closet, ready for use. The caregivers felt respected and the residents had options for their baths.

In addition, with this same nurse's support, nursing assistants who gained expertise in person-directed bathing of persons with dementia became the "bathing experts" in the facility. They assisted other caregivers to adopt this approach, helping to improve care on units for persons who were frail and in need of flexibility in their bathing routines.

Not all direct caregivers are skilled at working with people with dementia. Some need help dealing with care refusals or identifying and implementing alternate plans for bathing. In a transformed facility part of the supervisor's job is to educate, model, and support positive caregiving behaviors so that the medical and psychosocial needs of the residents are met. In addition, it is also necessary to identify where improvement is needed, set up a plan of correction, and give feedback in a way that motivates the caregiver.

Resources for Changing Roles

A major focus of person-directed care involves reexamining and redefining the roles of the nurse and the caregiver. There are a number of workshops and programs that have been developed to assist and support staff in making these role changes. One is called LEAP (Learn, Empower, Achieve, Produce, www.matherlifeways.com/re_leap.asp) developed by Anna Ortigara and others at Mather LifeWays, in Chicago, Illinois. Another is called Coaching Supervision, developed by Sara Joffe and others at Paraprofessional Health Institute in Philadelphia and New York City (2005, www.paraprofessional.org). Both teach skills such as active listening, presenting the problem,

EXHIBIT 12.4 Suggested Process for Moving From Rotating Assignments to Consistent Assignments

1. Call two meetings, one with all of the direct caregivers from the day shift and one with all direct caregivers from evening shift on a particular unit or household.
2. Begin the meeting by explaining that nursing homes that have switched to consistent assignment have been proven to improve quality of care and life for the residents and the quality of work life for the staff. Suggest that we pilot test consistent assignment and see how it works. Using a learning circle, ask them to express their feelings and concerns about making a change.
3. If there is consensus to try it, move forward. If not, set up a meeting for the following week and discuss it again. Explain the proposed process for change and that there would be a chance to re-evaluate how it is working in 3 months.
4. When you have reached a majority consensus and/or people are willing to try, move forward.
5. Place each resident's name on a Post-it note and place all of the Post-it notes on the wall.
6. Next, ask the group to rank each of the residents by degree of difficulty, with number 1 being relatively easy, number 3 in the middle, and number 5 being very difficult to care for (time consuming, emotionally draining, etc.). Let the direct caregivers discuss each resident and come to an agreement on the rankings. Write the rank on the resident's Post-it note.
7. Then, allow them to select their assignments. Assignments are fair when CNA assignments have similar total resident rankings. In other words, if one assignment has six residents and another has eight residents but the degree of difficulty rankings total 27 for both direct caregivers then the assignments are fair. Relationships with residents are important and also should be part of the decision-making process. The sequence of rooms is less important.
8. Meet every 3 months to re-examine that the assignments, based upon degree of difficulty, are still fair and that the relationships between resident and staff are still agreeable to both parties.

Adapted from RI QIO Quality Partners, 2006

and self-awareness that are important to be an effective supervisor.

TRANSFORMING BATHING CARE: CONTINUITY OF CAREGIVERS

Consistent Assignments vs. Rotation

Staffing patterns are crucial in determining the quality of the bathing experience. We have discussed the importance of having the same person doing the bathing. This can be accomplished in several ways and will likely require changes in the organization's procedures. One method is described in Exhibit 12.4.

Many facilities have switched to what is called consistent or permanent assignments. This means that a direct caregiver on each shift is assigned to care for the same group of people over time. This caregiver knows the needs and wishes of these residents, and their routines can be honored. On her days off, a consistent associate caregiver fills in. The idea is to have as few different caregivers as possible for each person. Other caregivers in the facility or the household (unit) will also need to know about the individual so they can fill in when needed. The primary caregiver provides information by word of mouth and also in the care plan.

Case Study

Here is a case study that illustrates a facility that has implemented the change necessary to individualize bathing:

Helen is consistently assigned to Mrs. Jonson, who is usually bathed on Saturday. However, this Saturday Helen is sick and Mrs. Jonson wishes to wait until Helen returns to get her shower. This wish is honored. The caregiver filling in invites another resident to shower instead to lighten the load for Helen when she returns. Helen will do her best to get Mrs. Jonson showered the day she returns, but if that is not possible she will negotiate with her, being sure that necessary parts are washed to prevent problems.

Case Discussion

In this facility person-directed bathing and teamwork are valued. Mrs. Jonson's wishes are more important than getting a bath on a designated day. Caregivers work together, adjusting their schedules, helping each other. Helen recognizes that Mrs. Jonson likes the routine they have worked out

> *in the shower where she is bathed with a no-rinse soap and is not sprayed with the hose. Helen also knows that she has the support of her supervisor, who will be more concerned about honoring Mrs. Jonson's wishes than whether she is bathed on a particular day. Because of the relationship they have built, Helen knows that Mrs. Jonson trusts she will do all she can to shower her when she returns and make it a pleasant experience.*

EXHIBIT 12.5 Benefits of Consistent Assignments: Caregiver Point of View

- Creating closer, more meaningful relationships with residents
- Easier to plan the workday
- Provides more job satisfaction
- Creates less staff turnover
- Caregivers who are not doing a good job become readily apparent
- Fewer items such as clothing, grooming articles, or assistive devices getting lost
- Families know who to ask for information
- Better relationships are formed with families

Many facilities appear confused about what is meant by consistent assignments. Some have stopped switching caregivers from unit to unit but still rotate the group of residents in their unit assignment. Others rotate care assignments after a month. These methods may be an improvement from the past but are not the level of consistency that best serves residents and are fast becoming outdated. There is general consensus and a growing body of literature (Bowers, 2003; Bowers, Esmond, & Jacobson, 2000; Burgio, Fisher, Fairchild, Scilley, & Hardin, 2004) that supports the concept of consistent assignments as a critical organizational element for creating person-directed care and lowering staff turnover.

Sometimes caregivers initially say they prefer the old rotating system to avoid getting "burned out" on residents who are not easy to work with. When a change toward more consistency in assignments is suggested, comments such as "I couldn't stand to take care of some of them for more than a week" are sometimes expressed. Facilities that have switched to permanent or consistent assignments find that different caregivers prefer different types of people. Allowing the caregivers to pick who is in their assignment usually works out well. In time, if they become frustrated with caring for someone, ways can be established for them to shift that person to another assignment.

Think about it. The goal is to create home, family, and relationship in care settings. How many of us in our own families have had moments when we wanted to "rotate" off the parenting or caregiver role and give it to someone else? Yet that is not what we do. We stay there and work things out as best we can as a family, drawing on all available resources. When there is a self-directed work team in an institutional setting, solutions evolve from team problem solving just as they do in well-functioning families. Almost without exception, people who live in care settings, as well as their families, prefer having permanently assigned staff who know and care

about them. So the effort spent on creating consistent assignments is worthwhile.

Direct caregivers who switch to consistent assignments generally come to prefer it. The benefits they identify are listed in Exhibit 12.5.

Problems can occur with consistent or permanent assignments. Caregivers may become very attached to certain persons. When these individuals become ill and die, caregivers may feel like they have lost a family member. Therefore, these situations need to be anticipated and addressed. For example, arrangements need to be made so staff can attend funerals. Some kind of ceremony or way of honoring deaths can be established within the facility. All staff need to know it is natural and acceptable to grieve these deaths. Sometimes a staff member can become too possessive of someone. Then, it is the role of the self-directed team or the nurse or other supervisor to help sort out what is best. From the resident's perspective, the departure of a favorite staff member can be a painful and difficult situation. Again, this situation needs to be anticipated. These problems grow out of caring. Wouldn't you rather be bathed by someone who cares rather than by someone who is just performing a task?

Specialized Bathing Staff

Another method used to create continuity is to have a caregiver, usually called a "bath aide," whose sole task is to bathe people. Because they do not have other care tasks, these caregivers often have a lot of flexibility in terms of time of day (within their assigned shift) or day of the week that bathing can be done. In addition, many bath aides take a great deal of pride in creating a pleasant experience for the person and are very skilled at their craft. Unless these individuals get pulled from their bathing duties because of staff call-ins or shortages, this method usually provides consistency in bathing.

In summary, there are many ways that staff can be assigned to bathe residents. The goal should be to have consistent and caring people with the ability to adjust the time of day, day of the week, and method to meet the person's wishes and changing needs.

Transforming Bathing Care: The Importance of Flexibility

The caregiver needs to have the decision-making authority to adjust to both the method and the frequency of bathing. This authority should be supported by changes in the organization's policy. An example of a person-directed policy related to bathing someone in the shower is in the Chapter Appendix. This policy clearly supports choice, preference, and making bathing a pleasant experience. How a person is bathed requires moment-by-moment decisions and, therefore, can't be dictated by inflexible, established bathing schedules. All the variations described in previous chapters should be considered viable bathing methods. These include such options as in-bed and in-room bathing, bathing in the shower, using a no-rinse soap, and dividing up the bathing into smaller tasks. In addition, physical and occupational therapists can be available to help figure out how to adapt the method of bathing and the environment to be more supportive.

Time of day and frequency also need to be flexible. Some facilities still awaken people for showers at 4:00–5:00 a.m. so that the night shift can "help" out the day shift's workload. Unless that is the resident's choice and custom to bathe at that hour, that practice is an excellent example of the task-oriented, industrial model of care. The bathing needs of all residents are not equal. It is clear that persons who experience incontinence, perspire heavily, or spill food require frequent freshening up for good health and skin care. However, washing the entire body and hair twice a week may be unnecessary. In several facilities in North Carolina and Oregon, many people were bathed only once a week for 3 months using a no-rinse soap solution and were not rinsed or washed with running water. No negative clinical effects from either reducing the number of baths or eliminating the running water were observed when they continued these practices on an ongoing basis after the research was completed.

Facilities might find it useful to question old patterns and rituals. Traditionally, care facilities assign a bath or shower by establishing a routine number of times a week it is to be done and randomly assigning residents to particular days of the week and time of day (shift). The most common routine appears to be twice-weekly baths or showers. This number is not based on any hard evidence but is a generally accepted standard of practice. Although some places have begun to re-evaluate this "sacred cow," it needs to be addressed in all facilities. Frequency of baths should be person-directed.

Doesn't it make more sense to look at an individual's preferences and needs to determine how and when bathing will occur? Some people may desire and need less frequent bathing while others may prefer to bathe daily. Meeting these wishes becomes more plausible with flexibility. Supervisors of direct caregivers need to re-examine existing bathing policies in light of the new evidence and allow responsible caregivers the autonomy and flexibility to create person-directed bathing.

HOW TO CHANGE THE CULTURE OF CARE IN YOUR FACILITY

Build Support for Change

The culture change movement encourages facilities to first become learning organizations that study and build inclusion of residents and all levels of caregiving staff in decisions. Support and commitment from administration as well as education, equipment, and consultation are critical for success. Many facilities form interdisciplinary culture change leadership teams to learn about and guide the overall culture change process. The administrator and director of nursing need to be part of this committee and attend the meetings, as do representatives from various departments, residents, family members, and direct care workers. Culture change or practice change cannot be imposed from the top down. Discussion and learning at all levels is needed for acceptance of new practices.

One useful tool for learning and building inclusion is the learning circle (see Exhibit 12.6, The Learning Circle). The learning circle is a tradition used in many settings and cultures to gather information and build a sense of community. It has been widely used by facilities working on transforming care (Norton, 2003). Basically, it involves a process where each person in the circle of

TABLE 12.6   The Learning Circle

Purpose of a Learning Circle:

- to give all a voice
- to create understanding
- to share decision making
- to solve problems
- to create a sense of community
- to give all a chance to be leaders.

Rules of the Learning Circle:

- Get in groups of 8–10 without a table
- Assign someone to be the facilitator
- The facilitator simply assures that no cross talk occurs until all are heard from
- The facilitator poses a question, topic, or problem
- Someone volunteers to start
- The group decides to go around circle either to the left or right
- If a person has nothing to say at her turn, she can pass
- After going all around the circle, the facilitator returns to people who passed to see if they now have something to add
- After all have had the opportunity to speak, the facilitator opens the conversation for general discussion.

8–12 has a chance to share how she feels about a topic, question, or problem that is presented to the group. All who wish to speak are heard before a general discussion begins. This creates an opportunity for the quiet person to talk and for those who tend to dominate conversations to be better listeners.

The reasons you have a circle, who attends, and the outcome will vary. At first, it may be used to build trust and to share opinions on topics such as current bathing practices. Later, it could be used to problem solve how to improve bathing for a particular person. Or, a quick circle could be used to decide how the workload will be divided when someone calls in sick. One household used it with residents to plan a party for a staff member who was getting married. Sometimes the learning circle results in a specific decision or plan and sometimes it provides a way to share thoughts or concerns.

When considering a change in bathing practices, separate learning circles for direct caregivers and residents allows both to feel free to discuss their bathing experiences openly. Residents could be asked how they feel about the way they are bathed and give suggestions for ways to improve. Caregivers could also discuss their concerns and ideas for improvements. Build your plans for change around the input you receive.

Transforming Care: Taking Action

The next step is to form a performance improvement bathing team to develop a plan of action. Members of the team might include nurses, direct caregivers, the in-service coordinator, the purchaser of supplies, at least one resident and family member, laundry, housekeeping, and perhaps maintenance, since all will be affected by bathing changes.

- *Look at your policies, procedures, and documentation.* Review policies and procedures. Does the bathing policy state that residents will be bathed or showered twice a week? Is it a "refusal" if the person is bathed in bed rather than taken to the shower? It is best to have a policy that simply states that hygiene needs will be met and addressed according to the person's preferences and changing needs. There is no required frequency or specific method for bathing in the federal nursing home regulations. If care plans simply state that hygiene needs will be met by a bed bath once a week, there is no need to document "refused shower." "Credit" is given for bathing regardless of the method used. Also, quarterly summaries should document what method is successful, or if not, how changes are made. Bathing procedures can be specified so they guide the caregivers through each step in a way that honors preferences and meets the needs of the person being bathed. An example of a procedure for showering is in the Appendix of this chapter.
- *Look at job descriptions.* Focus on language that emphasizes relationships and person-directed care (see Exhibit 12.7, Job Descriptions: Person-Directed Language).
- *Focus on exploring and trying different methods of bathing.* Try some of the techniques mentioned in this book, such as covering during the shower, washing the hair last, and using the no-rinse methods so you are familiar with them. Discuss these techniques during learning circles or care planning conferences. Gather data on behaviors that indicate discomfort during bathing and any changes that result from different techniques (see Appendix A, Measuring Success). Using different bathing methods is a fairly concrete and easy way to begin.
- *Create a plan for implementing person-directed bathing.* If your facility is new to the culture

EXHIBIT 12.7   Job Descriptions: Person-Directed Language

NURSE:

Person-Centered, Elder-Directed, Quality-Focused: Models and ensures that others are providing medical treatment in a manner that honors resident preferences and individuality. Demonstrates strong commitment to the highest clinical outcomes.

Leadership: Sees supervision of other staff as a role of service rather than as one of authority and seeks to support supervisees' ability to succeed. Willing to do any tasks needed, including those that may seem menial or unpleasant. When communicating with physician or other medical personnel advocates for resident preferences. Refrains from pressuring or manipulating residents into accepting medication or treatment for the sake of staff or facility convenience.

CERTIFIED NURSING ASSISTANT-CAREGIVER

Person-Centered, Elder-Directed, Quality-Focused: Caregivers observe and connect with residents in a way that gives them clear insights into each individual's preferences and concerns. Caregivers demonstrate the intention to strive for high efficiency while always respecting and preserving residents' personhood.

Adapted from the Household Matters Toolkit, Living & Working in Harmony, Integrated Human Resource System, courtesy of the Action Pact, Inc.

change journey or is a large facility, start small. Exhibit 12.8 describes a suggested process.

- *Address the larger, system issues that affect bathing.* When creating change, you may be encountering questions and obstacles related to frequency of bathing, staffing patterns, bathing equipment and supplies, and the role of the caregiver and supervisor. Clearly, changing the way staff think, feel about, and practice bathing influences many elements of the care system. It is important to address the big-picture issues as they emerge. Here are some to consider:

EXHIBIT 12.8   Plan for Implementing Person-Directed Bathing

- Pick the household or unit that you feel would be the most supportive. Factors to consider include the quality of the teamwork, the enthusiasm for new procedures, and the adequacy of resources available. It is also helpful if the household or unit already has consistent assignments.
- Create your quality improvement bathing team
- Create a budget if needed and request equipment and supplies
- Begin the learning process with the bathing team
  - Start by having a discussion with the direct caregivers and asking how they feel about the current approach to bathing
  - Have a similar discussion with residents
  - Look at and discuss videotape "Bathing Without a Battle" (see chapter 13, Resources)
  - Discuss the myths of bathing (chapter 1, Understanding the Battle)
- Have the team provide an inservice (see suggested outline in chapter 13,
- Innovative Approaches to Teach Person-Directed Bathing) to familiarize staff with plans/interventions
- Identify willing team members and have them practice any new methods or techniques with a volunteer resident who can provide them with feedback
- Select one resident (it is best to start with the simplest case)
- Decide what you want to change (develop specific goals), what success will look like, and how you will measure and document it (see Appendixes A, B, and C)
- Continue the trial-and-error process until your goals are achieved. Chapter 5, Selecting Person-Directed Solutions That Work, describes tools for identifying and measuring goals
- Document your revised, person-directed plan for bathing
- Repeat this process with another resident
- Set up a facility quality improvement program (see Appendix A, Measuring Success, for suggestions)
- Share your success with others through data and stories
- Have regular meetings of the bathing team to discuss progress and to solve problems

- *Be proactive with regulators (surveyors, protective service) and advocates.* A common concern expressed by providers is that the suggested bathing changes will not be seen positively by surveyors. It is best to take a proactive approach. Let surveyors know the positive things you are doing to improve practice. Remember, there is nothing in the federal regulations that mandates when, where, or how often people in care facilities are bathed. Show them the data you have gathered on comfort during bathing. Talk about specific techniques you have tried for persons who were upset during bathing. Ask them to share any questions or concerns. Be sure you have changed your policies and procedures to reflect person-directed bathing so there is no conflict. Since surveyors in many states are familiar with the bathing research and practices described here, many will be looking for evidence that you are working to make bathing as pleasant as possible for the individuals in your care.
- *Be proactive with families.* Another concern is that families will not be supportive of no-rinse methods of bathing. Let family members know your concerns about comfort during bathing and the efforts you are making to honor individual preferences. Assure family members of your commitment to quality care and good hygiene. Ask about prior bathing habits and ideas for comfortable bathing. Have your new "experts" provide a program for families to share examples of successes and solutions. You may wish to share with them the myths of bathing list (see chapter 1, Understanding the Battle) and show them parts of the "Bathing Without a Battle" video http://bathingwithoutabattle.unc.edu/.

Moving to person-directed bathing is a process. Policies, procedures, and roles may need to be changed. New practices may be adopted. It is important to gather data throughout the process and celebrate your successes. It will be a win-win for all.

BATHING AT HOME

The organizational issues for families caring for persons with dementia at home are different than those for caregivers in facilities. Usually, fewer people are caring for the person at home, thus providing care and continuity in existing relationships. Being a solitary caregiver can be tiring and overwhelming, causing stress, anger, and frustration. The bathing experience may feel like a battle, particularly if the person resists your efforts to help. Taking care of yourself is as important as taking care of your family member with dementia as explained in chapter 14, Taking Care of Yourself: Strategies for Caregivers.

Sometimes family members or friends wanting to be helpful may give advice or criticism without recognizing the complexity of the situation. What you may need from members of your family and friendship network are:

- Someone you can talk to, who is a good listener rather than advice giver
- Someone to provide concrete help with specific tasks and activities
- Someone to provide occasional respite from caregiving.

For example, a friend or other family member could do the shopping, pick up medications, take over some household chores, or provide assistance with personal care activities such as bathing. Your ability to reach out and ask specifically for assistance is very important to your health. If your health fails or you become overwhelmed, your ability to provide care at home will be compromised.

Thinking Creatively About Bathing

Family members also need to examine their own myths about keeping people clean. Holding onto the belief that you must have a shower or tub bath to get clean limits options and creates unnecessary, upsetting situations. For many reasons, bathing can be overwhelming for the person. Many of the ideas discussed in chapters 3, 4, and 5 are very adaptable to the home setting. Here are some additional ideas to consider.

Consider Options Other Than the Shower or Tub

The numerous no-rinse products that are currently on the market and presented in this book can be very useful to family or in-home caregivers. One family reported that it divided the body into seven parts and washed a different part each day of the week. This kept the person clean without causing the person to be overwhelmed by the demands of a shower or a total body wash at one time.

Shared Bathing

Sometimes spouses or partners find it helpful and easy to join the person in the shower and bathe together. If this is an acceptable option for you, it can provide a time of caring and intimacy that both of you will find pleasurable.

Adult Children as Caregivers

When an adult child takes on the role of bathing a parent, it can be emotionally difficult. At first the change of roles may feel awkward and uncomfortable. Using humor can often make the situation easier for all. There can be rewards, too, for both the parent and adult child. Assisting with bathing provides a way to "give back" to a parent who may prefer to have a family member rather than a stranger assist with such an intimate activity.

Sometimes, if the person with dementia doesn't recognize the adult child or thinks he/she is the spouse, the person may make sexual comments or advances that feel inappropriate or distressing. Family members have chosen to stop assisting with bathing because of their distress related to such behaviors. These actions need to be looked at in the context of the illness that is causing the disorientation and disinhibition. Persons with dementia may say and do things that are completely out of character for them because their "censor functions" no longer work. Clarifying who you are and setting limits can be helpful in some cases. For example, you could say: "Dad, I'm your daughter. Please stop."

Using Outside Resources to Help

Hiring someone to come into the home to provide assistance with bathing, perhaps along with providing respite to you as the caregiver, can be very beneficial. If you feel the person may be resistant to having someone else help with personal care, start out with the hired caregiver coming in and getting to know the person first. Look for someone with experience working with persons who have dementia. You are looking for a caregiver who can help get the person to say "yes" and adapt bathing to the needs of your family member. For example, some hired in-home caregivers report that they have bathed people quite well while they were sitting in a recliner.

The bathrooms in the home may be small and may or may not be adapted to meet changing physical and emotional needs. Chapter 10, The Physical Environment of the Bathing Room, has good information about how to adapt the bathroom to make it a friendlier, safer place.

CONCLUSION

Changing the beliefs and practices about bathing can be a challenge, especially in organizational settings. Even at home most caregivers have certain ways they provide care, and changing can be hard to do. This chapter describes the key concepts and steps for creating change in bathing approaches. Moving to person-directed bathing can serve as a model for creating systemwide culture change, creating organizations that emphasize choice, relationship, and dignity that results in improved care and greater job satisfaction.

It is important to build inclusion and support for change throughout the organization. Many facilities have found it helpful to create culture change leadership teams to study and guide organizational changes. In addition, smaller bathing teams may be useful in guiding specific practice changes related to bathing. Piloting change can be helpful and is one way to "grow" in-house experts who can serve as role models for their peers. Gathering data throughout the process can provide specific information for quality improvement.

Family members who provide care at home can use many of the ideas on how to individualize the bathing experience. They too need to get free of the myth that it takes a lot of water to get someone clean. They also need to reach out to others when they are feeling overwhelmed and at a loss for how to address bathing needs.

Providing person-directed care fosters trust, a very real commodity in the caregiving relationship. When caregivers are put in the position of bathing someone against her will, it destroys trust that takes time and energy to develop. Caregivers may "harden their hearts" and turn bathing into just a task to be done because it is too painful to continually do something that the person being cared for doesn't want done or perceives as an assault. Such experiences can lead to caregiver frustration, burnout, and turnover. For this reason and others discussed in this book, people should not be bathed against their will unless there is a compelling health reason. To do so is abuse. Although changing bathing practices may not be easy in all cases, the benefits for the relationship are worth it!

REFERENCES

Baker, B. (2007). *Old age in a new age: The promise of transformative nursing homes.* Nashville, TN: Vanderbilt University Press.

Bowers, B. J. (2003). Turnover reinterpreted: CNAs talk about why they leave. *Journal of Gerontological Nursing, 29*(3), 36–44.

Bowers, B. J., Esmond, S., & Jacobson, N. (2000). The relationship between staffing and quality in long-term care facilities: Exploring the views of nurse aides. *Journal of Nursing Care Quality, 14*(4), 55–64.

Burgio, L. D., Fisher, S. E., Fairchild, J. K., Scilley, K., & Hardin, M. (2004). Quality of care in the nursing home: Effects of staff assignment and work shift. *The Gerontologist, 44*(3), 368–377.

Fox, N. (2007). *The journey of a lifetime: Leadership pathways to culture change in long-term care.* Milwaukee, WI: Action Pact Inc.

Norton, L. (2003). The power of circles: Using a familiar technique to promote culture change. *Journal of Social Work in Long-Term Care, 2*(3/4), 285–292.

Paraprofessional Health Institute. (2005). *Coaching supervision: Introductory skills for supervisors in home and residential care.* New York: National Clearinghouse on the Direct Care Workforce.

Seavey, D. (2004). *The cost of frontline turnover in long-term care.* Better Jobs Better Care Practice and Policy Report, 1–3. Washington, DC: Institute for the Future of Aging Services, American Association of Homes and Services for the Aging.

Shields, S., & Norton, L. (2006). *In pursuit of a sunbeam: A practical guide to transformation from institution to household.* Milwaukee, WI: Action Pact Inc.

Shields, S., Norton, L., Bump, L., & Maben, P. (2006). *Household matters toolkit, integrated human resources system.* Manhattan, KS: Retirement Foundation d/b/a/ Meadowlark Hills Retirement Community (available at www.pioneernetwork.net).

Thomas, W. (1999). *The Eden Alternative handbook: The art of building human habitats.* Sherburne, NY: Summer Hill.

Thomas, W. (2004). *What are old people for? How elders will save the world.* Acton, MA: VanderWyk & Burnham.

RESOURCE

Bathing Without a Battle—CD/Video
http://bathingwithoutabattle.unc.edu/

APPENDIX

Community Name

Preparing to Bathe a Resident

Procedure Number: 11.03.01   42 CFR: 483.25(a)

Date Approved: F Tag: 310

Supersedes: State Reg.

                                                                                 MDS 2.0: G.2

Employees Responsible: Licensed nurses and caregivers

Policy: Team members who assist residents with bathing will focus on making the bathing experience enjoyable for the resident.

Procedure:

1. Review the information about bathing found on the resident's preferences sheet in the resident preference notebook.

   a. Time of day resident prefers to bathe.
   b. Where does the resident prefer to be bathed?
   c. Type of bath resident prefers.
      i Tub bath/whirlpool
      ii Shower
      iii Sponge bath
      iv Towel bath in own bed
   d. Does the resident prefer to undress and dress in his/her bedroom or in the spa?
   e. Does the resident have a preference for a bathing product or products to be used during the bath?
   f. If resident enjoys music while bathing, what music does he/she prefer?
   g. How long does the resident like to remain in the tub or shower?
   h. Does the resident want to avoid getting his/her face wet?

2. Record on the resident preferences form any new information you find out about the resident's bathing preferences.
3. If you are bathing a resident for the first time, talk with the resident and confirm his/her preferences.
4. When the resident is unable to provide you with information about his/her preferences, talk with another team member or a family member about the resident's preferences and successful approaches to assist the resident in enjoying the bathing experience.
5. As you prepare to bathe a resident, focus on the resident and his/her preferences rather than on the task of bathing.
6. Ensure that the room in which the resident is to be bathed is warm.
7. Gather all the supplies and equipment you will need before approaching the resident.

Shields, Norton, Bump, & Maben (2006), courtesy of Manhattan Retirement Foundation d/b/a Meadowlark Hills Retirement Community

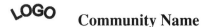 **Community Name**

Assisting a Resident With a Shower Bath

Procedure Number: 11.03.02
Date Approved:
Supersedes:

42 CFR: 483.25(a)
F Tag: 310
State Reg.
MDS 2.0 G.2

Employees Responsible: Licensed nurses and caregivers

Equipment:

- Shower chair or gurney if appropriate for resident
- Towels and washcloths
- Soap and/or shower gel of resident's choice
- Moisturizing lotion for skin
- Shampoo of resident's choice if needed
- Change of clothing or bathrobe for resident

Procedure:

1. If this is the first time you have assisted the resident with a shower, review the resident preference form in the resident preference notebook.
2. Bathing should be a comforting and relaxing time for the resident. Adjust the procedure to meet the individual needs and preferences of the resident.
3. Check spa to ensure:

    a. The auxiliary heating system is turned on and the room is at a comfortable temperature for the resident.
    b. Adequate supplies of towels and washcloths are available.

4. Gather the resident's personal bathing items such as shampoo, shower gel, and moisturizing lotion as requested by resident.
5. The resident preference form should indicate whether the resident prefers to be undressed and dressed in the spa or in his/her own bedroom.

    a. If the resident wishes to dress and undress in the bathing room, gather clothing according to resident's preferences.
    b. If the resident wishes to undress and dress in his/her bedroom, assist the resident into a heavy bathrobe.

6. Assist the resident to the bathing room. Place occupied sign on door to spa.
7. If resident enjoys music while bathing, place CD of his/her choice in CD player.
8. Talk to resident quietly during the bath. Explain what you are doing. If the resident appears anxious, take time to recognize his/her anxiety. If resident becomes upset, stop the bath.
9. Pull privacy curtain so that resident is not visible if door to room is opened.
10. Offer to assist the resident to toilet. If fecal material is present in anal area, apply gloves, wipe with toilet paper, and then with a wet washcloth. Remove gloves, dispose in waste container, and wash hands.
11. Assist the resident to remove clothing. Some residents will appreciate a towel over their shoulders.

12. If transferring to a bath chair ensure that resident's feet will touch the floor when seated and that the seat is padded for comfort.
13. Cover front of body with a large bath towel.
14. Place soap and shampoo on shelf in shower.
15. Turn water on slowly. Adjust temperature. Allow resident to test water for comfortable temperature.
16. Offer the resident a wet washcloth with soap to wash his/her face. If resident is unable to perform this task, wash the resident's face, neck, and ears gently. Rinse washcloth and wipe soap off face.
17. If washing the resident's hair in the shower, offer the resident a dry washcloth to hold over eyes, lean head back to wet hair. Try to keep shower spray away from resident's face.
18. Remove towel from shoulders, lower towel over upper half of body, and wash trunk, back, underarms, and arms. Rinse off soap using spray. Keep water from splashing onto resident's face.
19. Replace towel on shoulders and upper half of body.
20. Remove lower half of towel from legs, wash legs and feet.
21. Offer a clean washcloth to resident to wash perineum.
22. If resident is unable to wash perineum don gloves and clean perineum.

   a. For women residents, wash front to back using a clean portion of washcloth each time.
   b. For men residents cleanse penis and then anal area.
   c. Use spray to rinse area.

23. Using a dry towel, pat dry skin. Observe for discolorations, open areas, and other changes in the resident's skin.
24. Be sure to dry between and under skin folds including underneath arms, breasts, abdomen, groin creases, perineal and rectal areas, and between toes.
25. Apply moisturizer to skin as desired by resident.
26. Assist resident into robe or to dress in street clothes or sleepwear. Groom resident according to his/her preferences.
27. Return resident to bedroom or to place of resident's choice within the household.
28. Place used towels and wash clothes into laundry hamper.
29. Spray shower chair or gurney with detergent/disinfectant. Wipe dry.
30. Return resident's personal bathing supplies and other belongings to his/her bedroom.
31. Report to licensed nurse any observations of the resident's skin or other concerns noted during the bathing procedure.

Shields, Norton, Bump, & Maben (2006), courtesy of Manhattan Retirement Foundation d/b/a Meadowlark Hills Retirement Community

CHAPTER 13

Interactive Approaches to Teach Person-Directed Bathing

Joyce H. Rasin, Joanne Rader, Ann Louise Barrick

Two of the fundamental values in the bathing approach discussed in previous chapters are person-directed bathing and the importance of the relationship between the care provider and the care receiver. These values are also important in the approach to training care providers. In person-directed bathing, the care provider recognizes that the care recipient has preferred ways of getting clean. Instructors in a training situation must also be aware that participants have preferred ways of learning. Likewise, the interaction between instructor and participant is just as important as the care provider–care receiver interaction. The effective instructor is sensitive and responds to the needs of the participant. Furthermore, responses are influenced by feedback received from the participant. This chapter will discuss how to create a supportive learning environment, suggest teaching strategies that are appropriate for different learning styles, and describe the necessary components of clinical learning.

CREATING A SUPPORTIVE LEARNING ENVIRONMENT

The instructor must take the lead in setting the tone for the class in order to maximize participants' motivation to learn and share. A positive learning environment is emotionally and physically comfortable and communicates respect for participants. It recognizes that the participants also have a lot to teach each other and the instructor.

Creating Comfort

Icebreakers and warm-up exercises are useful for creating a comfortable learning environment. Even when participants know each other, warm-up activities can encourage involvement and interaction. They help participants get to know each other and the instructor, and they establish the emotional climate for the class. One good warm-up exercise is to ask participants to name one thing they would like to learn during the class. The instructor can review these expectations with the group and explain how the group's learning goals fit into the planned material. Knowing the concerns of the group can also help the instructor adapt the information to the needs of the group as much as possible. If participants have learning goals that will not be addressed in the class, these goals might be good suggestions for developing future classes.

Communicating Respect

It is also important for the instructor to communicate respect for participants at all times. A basic rule of thumb to follow is that there is never a dumb question or response. Accept and value all responses that are made in the spirit of learning. The response may contain incorrect information, but the instructor can acknowledge the participation and clarify the information. Active listening is the most important communication skill for demonstrating respect, acceptance, and interest. It is also important to be aware of nonverbal behavior that may communicate a lack of attention, such as glancing away, interrupting a participant, and failing to make eye contact. Keep in mind, however, that participants' cultural background must be taken into account when determining what nonverbal behavior communicates interest or disinterest.

Motivating the Adult Learner

Individuals need to be motivated if learning is to occur. This poses a dilemma. Many inservice classes are mandatory. Although people can be forced to attend, they may not be motivated to learn. The instructor has to work harder initially to engage the reluctant participant with low motivation. Consider the following factors when attempting to enhance participants' motivation.

Usefulness of Information

The participant must see a use for the material presented. Adults need to know why they should learn new information. If the usefulness is not apparent, interest may be low. Capture the attention of the participants in the beginning of the session by describing how the topic relates to the skills needed for their work. Many care providers find that bathing individuals with dementia is difficult and problematic, so one effective strategy would be to ask the participants what problems they experience when bathing residents.

Elicit discussion of care providers' prior experiences and link something from their experience to some new piece of information. Asking the care providers how they have made bathing more pleasant for people is another good starting point that acknowledges them as experts and establishes that the instructor recognizes this. Although this is most desirable it may not always be possible. Some old experiences should not be reinforced. Your staff may have been involved in activities in previous employment that reflect old practice standards or just misinformation. Resistance to accepting new information can be due to a negative evaluation of its usefulness based on prior experiences. Knowing about divergent viewpoints provides the trainer with an excellent opportunity to engage the learner in some problem solving and show how it can be currently applied.

Caregiver Wisdom

Most care aides were taught to start washing from the top (the hair) down. This just upsets people with dementia so I go with what is least upsetting to them, maybe their face, maybe their feet. We have to teach that it is OK to alter how you wash people to meet their needs.
Kathy House, CNA, Fairlawn Good Samaritan Health
Center, Gresham, OR

Applicability

The information needs to be not only useful but also readily applicable to specific work situations. Motivation to learn increases when adult participants have a problem to solve. They want to know how information can be used with specific real-life problems and prefer that which is concrete and practical. Providing active learning exercises such as role-plays and learning circles (see next section) clearly demonstrates the applicability of the material and increases learner participation. Furthermore, active learning exercises are most appropriate for teaching a process such as bathing.

Incentives

Incentives can be both psychological and tangible. Emphasize that learning about person-directed bathing will make the experience more pleasurable for both the care provider and the care recipient. Tangible incentives such as refreshments and door prizes also increase interest. The incentives don't have to be costly. Most participants appreciate simply having a beverage or small door prize. Multicolored ink pens, pocket tablets, and hand lotion are useful and inexpensive, and they can be tied to some aspect of the training. Make the process of distributing the prizes fun, so participants associate a pleasurable experience with learning.

Positive Feelings

Clearly communicating the usefulness of the material, providing an opportunity to apply the material successfully, and providing incentives for learning will help participants feel positive about their experience. Positive feelings are very powerful motivators for learning and contribute to a participant's feelings of self-confidence and competence.

COMPONENTS OF CLINICAL TEACHING

Acquiring new skills can be broken into two components—obtaining information about the skill and supervised practice to become competent in the skill. Although both components are needed for proficiency, continuing education programs tend to emphasize only the knowledge component. This section focuses on

---

methods for providing information as well as the role of supervised practice.

Providing Information

Individuals acquire new information and skills in different ways. As an instructor, your participants will have different learning needs. One teaching method will not be suitable for all participants. Just as the care provider must have an assortment of approaches to use when working with a care receiver, the instructor should know multiple techniques for teaching and the range of possible learning needs in order to individualize teaching. In this section, specific teaching strategies are described.

Teaching Strategies

Lecture—This method is most frequently used in a classroom setting. It allows the instructor to provide a lot of information at one time to a large number of people. One negative aspect of lecture is that participant participation is limited, which prevents participants from learning to problem solve. Also, remembering lecture information is generally difficult unless participants are taking notes.

Visual Aids—When you don't have the real thing, because of cost or unavailability, drawings, photographs, overheads, or models can be substituted. These can be very effective when accompanied by clear explanations. Combining visual aids with lecture (i.e., illustrated lecture) is an effective way to provide lots of information in an organized manner while maintaining participants' attention and enhancing their ability to learn the material.

Audiovisual Aids—Materials such as videotapes or slides are a good supplement to other methods such as lecture or discussion. When a demonstration or role-play is not feasible, videotape or slides provide a good substitute. The "Bathing Without a Battle" CD and videotape are also excellent resources to augment the teaching of person-directed bathing and to enhance learning (see resources in Chapter Appendix). Be sure to take time to plan how the audiovisuals will be used within the lecture, especially when using them for the first time. Rehearse with the equipment and your notes so that you can do both smoothly. Videotapes can be used in place of an instructor when trying to reach staff members who are not available when the

class is taught (e.g., due to sickness, day off, another shift). However, if the staff has no opportunity to have questions answered and concerns clarified, learning and proper implementation can be compromised.

Discussion—Either lecture or videotapes may be used to elicit questions that lead to discussion.

Discussion gives participants an opportunity to exchange ideas. The interchange of ideas among participants provides substantial benefits to individual participants, including learning from the experiences of others and sharing different perspectives on the application of materials.

Learning Circle—The learning circle is a leveling technique that encourages quiet people to speak, talkative people to listen, and everyone to share in making decisions and finding solutions. Participants observe, interpret, and experience their own feelings about an issue and broaden their perspectives by considering the many viewpoints of others around them. Circles are most effective when they become a way of life in the nursing facility and everyone takes turns facilitating (Norton, 2003).

Demonstration—In a demonstration, you show and explain the steps of a task to the learner (e.g., covered massage bed bath or transferring) or show how to use a piece of equipment (e.g., bath chair). Because the learner uses both vision and hearing, memory and understanding are enhanced. The following steps are suggested for preparing a demonstration:

- Obtain all of the items that you will use and make sure all equipment you plan to use is working properly before the demonstration.
- Make sure everyone can see and hear you clearly from any location in the room.
- Before you start the demonstration, summarize what you will be doing.
- List each step in sequence.
- Talk through each step.
- If possible, allow each participant to perform the task (i.e., return demonstration).

Role-plays—Role-plays will help participants learn the person-directed bathing approach. Person-directed bathing means the caregiver has to be comfortable trying different approaches. Role-playing gives the learner a chance to think on the spot and practice different approaches in a safe environment. The trainer assists the learner in developing problem-solving skills. The following steps are suggested for developing a role-play:

- Write a description of a bathing scenario. This could be a combination of some past experiences.
- Describe the characteristics of the care provider and the care recipient.
- Brief each participant on his/her role individually.
- Allow the scene to evolve for 5–10 minutes. The length of time will vary with the participants.
- If the participants are shy or get stuck, ask the rest of the class to provide suggestions.

Case Study—Provide a written description of a situation that the caregivers might actually experience. This should be a realistic example, one in which the learner could imagine himself/herself. The instructor can then involve all participants in problem solving and identifying possible solutions.

Matching Teaching Strategies to Learning Styles of Participants

The instructor needs to decide which strategy is appropriate for the type of material being presented and the learning needs of the participants. The most effective approach for trying to use teaching strategies that match the learning style of all participants in the class is to employ a variety of approaches. The diversity of techniques will improve teaching the person-directed bathing approach since they will capture the interest of participants in different ways and reinforce material that is important to learn. At the end of this chapter, you will find examples of how lecture, discussion, demonstration, case studies, role-play, and visual aids can be employed to teach the components of person-directed bathing.

Supervised Practice

If skills that were learned in the classroom are not practiced, they will quickly be forgotten. A care provider might be reluctant to perform a new skill independently until he/she can develop both competence and confidence. Supervised practice fosters accurate mastery of skills because the care provider has the opportunity to perform the task or skill under the watchful eye of an experienced provider. Peers working as mentors/coaches can perform this role. The purpose of the clinical mentor or coach is to help the mentee apply the new skill in the clinical setting. The mentor should initially model the appropriate behaviors and then provide guidance as the novice tries out the new skill. The ideal mentor/coach is an expert in both clinical practice and in teaching clinical skills. Specifically, the mentor/ coach should be comfortable and competent with using a person-directed bathing approach and should be able to teach these skills to an adult learner. Skills needed by trainers include the ability to stimulate motivation and confidence and to present the material in a variety of teaching strategies. Acquiring the necessary training skills requires that new mentors/coaches also initially receive mentoring.

Caregiver Wisdom

As a designated mentor, I talk with the new aide before we go in. I explain a little about who the person is, what he/she likes and doesn't like, and the method of bathing that works best and why. Then I go in and demonstrate how to do it. After, I check to see if the aide has any questions. The next time, I help the aide set up and let him/her begin, and then I see how the aide is doing. If the aide needs assistance, I role model how to resolve the situation. If the aide seems comfortable, I step back. I make sure I give the aide feedback about how well he/she is doing.

Beth Parker, CNA, Marian Estates, Sublimity, OR

SUMMARY

The instructor is responsible for creating a supportive and comfortable learning environment for participants. To motivate adult participants, it is important to:

- clearly communicate the usefulness of the material
- demonstrate the applicability of the material in everyday situations
- provide incentives for learning
- engender participants with positive feelings such as confidence and competence.

The instructor should be familiar with a variety of different teaching strategies that are appropriate for participants' different learning needs and styles. Finally, clinical teaching should provide both useful information and supervised practice to help participants develop skillful approaches to bathing.

REFERENCE

Norton, L. (2003). The power of circles: Using a familiar technique to promote culture change. *Journal of Social Work in Long-Term Care, 20*(3–4).

RESOURCES

Bathing Without a Battle—CD/Video
http://bathingwithoutabattle.unc.edu/

Equipment: See chapter 11.

Videotape: Solving Bathing Problems in Persons With Alzheimer's Disease and Related Dementia by Phillip Sloane, Ann Louise Barrick, and Vanessa Horn. To order contact Health Professions Press at 1-888-337-8808 or its Web site: http://www.healthpropress.com/store/sloane-TN10/index.htm

APPENDIX

LEARNING PROGRAMS FOR ADMINISTRATORS, FAMILIES, NURSING ASSISTANTS, AND NURSING SUPERVISORS

Learning programs can be developed to meet the needs of administrators, nurse supervisors, direct caregivers (nursing assistants), and family caregivers. Use the following list of topics to tailor a learning program specifically for these targeted audiences (Table 13.1).

USING TEACHING STRATEGIES IN TRAINING

This section provides examples of how to apply the principles discussed earlier in this chapter to the teaching of the content presented in this book. Three exercises are described that teach the foundational concepts of empathy and triggers of distressed care receiver behavior. These exercises involve miniscripted role-play and discussion. A sample module for in-room bathing is also provided that integrates the teaching strategies of minilectures, discussion, demonstration, return demonstration, case studies, and visual aids.

Exercise 13.1—Empathy

Purpose: The purpose of this exercise is to help the participants appreciate the feelings of persons who are dependent and who have dementia.

Learning Objectives: At the end of this exercise, the participant will:

- Understand how care recipients might feel when being bathed
- Understand how care recipients' feelings might lead to challenging behaviors.

Instructor Preparation:

- Copy 13.1 Directions for Care Recipients and Caregivers (Appendix)

TABLE 13.1 Outline of Training for Bathing Persons With Dementia

Topic	Target Audience			
	DCG	NRS	FAM	ADM
Providing flexible bathing opportunities for patients and staff		X	X	X
Promoting teamwork in the provision of personal care		X		X
Problem-solving techniques that reduce agitation during bathing	X	X	X	
Communicating with the Alzheimer's patient	X	X	X	X
Transfer techniques	X	X	X	
Tips on successful in-room bathing	X	X	X	
Tips on successful showering	X	X	X	
Tips on successful tub bathing	X	X	X	
Equipment that can assist in bathing difficult patients		X	X	X

DCG = direct caregivers (e.g., nursing assistants); NRS = nurse supervisors; FAM = families; ADM = administrators

- Prepare one baggie for every two participants by putting a moist wipe in a baggie.
- If blackboard is not available, obtain flip chart, whiteboard, or some other portable writing surface.

Instructor:

- *We are going to do an exercise involving a caregiver and a care recipient. Please divide up into pairs. One person will be the care recipient, the other person will be the caregiver. I will give you directions that will tell you exactly what to do or say.*
- Give the following directions to the care recipients.

Care recipients—Directions

Stay seated

You can't talk

Put your hands behind your back

Try to do what you are told to do

Close your eyes now and keep them closed

After the "care recipients" have read the directions and closed their eyes, give the following written directions to the "caregivers" in a slide, on the flip chart, or on the board.

"Caregivers," after you read these directions, you may begin.

Caregiver—Directions

Take the wipe out of the baggie

Mumble, "Need to get this done. Hurry up!"

Touch your partner on the neck with the wipe

Tug at her clothes

Wipe her arm

Instructor:

- After the caregivers wipe the care recipient's arms, stop the role-play.
- Ask the participants to place the wipe back into the baggie for disposal.
- Ask the following questions to the care recipient and write responses on the blackboard or portable writing surface:

  - *How did it feel to be the care recipient?*
  - *What were your concerns?*
  - *What did you want to do?*

Ask the caregivers:

- *How did it feel to be the caregiver?*
- *What were your concerns?*
- *What did you want to do?*

Ask all students:

- *What are the similarities in the feelings, concerns, behaviors? Differences?*
- *What would you do to make this bathing experience more pleasant for the care recipient?*

Instructor: *This exercise was an exaggeration to make a point. However, persons who have dementia may be surprised, confused, upset, and frightened during bathing.*

- *Who have you bathed that gets upset?*
- *What have you tried that has helped?*

Wrap-up:

- *How would you summarize the potential feelings of a care recipient when a caregiver behaves like the caregivers in the exercise we did today?*
- *What can you do to help care recipients feel less upset?*
- *What have we discussed today that you can use with the persons for whom you care?*

Role-play can be stressful for students. In the next set of exercises you as the instructor will take the active role so the focus is on you. The critique is of the instructor's "role-play," not the student's.

Exercise 13.2—Physical and Emotional Triggers of Behavior, or "Why Is She Acting That way?" (Based on the case, "Adapting to Personal Factors," in chapter 4, "Assessing Behaviors")

Purpose: The purpose of this exercise is to help the participant identify and discuss the personal causes of some verbal and nonverbal distress behaviors of persons with dementia.

Learning Objectives:

- Identify verbalizations of distress made by persons with dementia during bathing
- Identify nonverbal behavior during bathing that indicates distress
- Discuss potential meanings of these verbalizations and behaviors.

Instructor Preparation:

- Read chapter 4, "Assessing Behaviors," and Table 4.1, "Different Expressions of Concern During Bathing," for a discussion of the relationship of verbal and nonverbal distress behaviors and pain, feeling lack of control, anxiety/fear, and cold.
- Copy Table 4.1 for students.
- Copy 13.2 directions (Appendix).
- If blackboard is not available, obtain flip chart, whiteboard, or some other portable writing surface.
- Bring a shower chair to the classroom.

Instructor:

- *We are going to examine the behaviors of some care recipients when getting a shower and discuss some causes for these behaviors.*
- *I will be Mrs. Peters, a person in the early stages of dementia. It is 10 a.m., so I am dressed, I have finished breakfast, and I am sitting in the community room. Would someone volunteer to be the caregiver? You will just have to read from a script. I would like everyone to listen and observe what Mrs. Peters says or does. Our focus is on Mrs. Peters.*
- Distribute the following script (Appendix) to the volunteer caregiver.

Scene 13.2A—Script

Caregiver: "Hi, Mrs. Peters, it is time for your bath. Let's go to the bathroom."

Mrs. Peters (instructor): "No, I have already had my bath."

Caregiver: "You have not had your bath yet, Mrs. Peters. Come on, it won't take long." Mrs. Peters (say a little louder): "I told you I had a bath!"

Caregiver: "Mrs. Peters, you are dirty. Don't you want to get nice and clean?"

Mrs. Peters: "I am not dirty! I already had a bath and I am NOT going to take a second one! Leave me alone!" (shake your fist at the caregiver)

Instructor:

- *Let's talk about how Mrs. Peters behaved and what she said. First, what did Mrs. Peters do that indicated she was distressed?* Help participants describe both verbal and nonverbal behavior.

  - *What made the behavior worse?*
  - *What do you think caused these behaviors?*

- Introduce the term "triggers of behavior"

  - Discuss personal needs and capabilities of care recipient as triggers (refer to Table 4.1)
  - Discuss possible triggers for Mrs. Peters

    - Dementia-related factors—memory and judgment

      - Didn't remember she had not bathed

    - Felt losing control

      - Not given a choice
      - Offended by suggestion she was dirty
      - Felt she had to defend herself

- *In the next scene, another caregiver has Mrs. Peters, the care recipient, sitting in a shower chair in the shower room. Could I have another volunteer caregiver?* Thank the first volunteer caregiver. *I will be Mrs. Peters.*

- Give the directions for scene 13.2B (Appendix) to the volunteer caregiver.

Scene 13.2B—Directions

Caregiver: Pretend you are washing Mrs. Peters's arm, lifting it to wash her underarm and bending her arm at the elbow.

Mrs. Peters (instructor): Cry and say "stop, stop" when your arm is lifted or the elbow is bent.

Instructor:

- *Why might Mrs. Peters be crying and saying stop?*

Guide the discussion to include the possibility of pain and/or feeling lack of control.

- *What verbal and nonverbal behaviors are clues to these feelings?*
- *What could you do to help Mrs. Peters be more comfortable?*

The third scene continues with Mrs. Peters. Give the directions for scene 13.2C (Appendix) to the volunteer caregiver.

Scene 13.2C—Directions

Caregiver: Continue to pretend to wash Mrs. Peters.

Mrs. Peters (instructor): Holler "Help, help." Look distressed and shiver like you are cold.

Instructor:

- *Why might Mrs. Peters be hollering "help" and shivering?*
- Guide the discussion to the possibility that Mrs. Peters is anxious or fearful and cold.
- *What behaviors suggest these feelings?*
- *What could you do to make Mrs. Peters more comfortable?*

Wrap-up:

- *Let's summarize. What are some of the feelings and physical factors that can trigger care recipient-distressed behaviors during bathing?*
- *Tell me how you will use something we discussed today when you are bathing someone.*
- *We have discussed how the care recipient's feelings and physical condition can trigger distressed behavior. In the next exercise we will look at the importance of caregiver behaviors in the relationship between the care recipient and the caregiver.*

Exercise 13.3—Caregiver Behaviors as Triggers

Purpose: The purpose of this exercise is to recognize the impact of the caregiver's approach on care recipient behavior.

Learning Objectives:

At the end of these exercises, the participants will:

- Identify caregiver behaviors that can trigger distressed behaviors by care recipients
- Describe caregiver behaviors that can facilitate the caregiver–care recipient relationship.

Instructor Preparation:

- Read section "Consider Relationship/Interpersonal Factors" in chapter 4, "Assessing Behaviors"
- Copy the directions for the care recipient and caregiver (Appendix)
- Copy handout, "Caregiver Behaviors as Triggers" (Appendix)
- If blackboard is not available, obtain a flip chart, whiteboard, or some other portable writing surface.

Instructor:

- *We have talked previously about how pain, cold, or fear can trigger distressed behavior like yelling "no" or "stop," hitting, and shivering. Sometimes we as caregivers can also trigger distressed behavior by how we behave or talk to persons with dementia. During this exercise I will be Caregiver Robin. I need two volunteers. One will be a caregiver working with me and the other will be*

Mrs. Baker, the care recipient. Each volunteer will get written directions about what to say. It will just be a couple of sentences. Who will volunteer?
- Distribute the directions (Appendix) to the volunteers who will be Mrs. Baker and the second caregiver.

Scene 13.3—Directions

Mrs. Baker, the care recipient:

Every few seconds say "I'm cold!," "I already had a bath." No matter what Caregiver Robin says, repeat "I'm cold." When Caregiver Robin tries to lift your arm, pull it back, saying "No, no, no!" and raise your hand and say "I'm going to hit you!"

Scene 13.3—Directions

Second Caregiver: You will be helping Caregiver Robin give Mrs. Baker a shower by just holding her arm. Caregiver Robin will be talking to you. Just appear to be interested by nodding your head and saying "uh huh."

Scene 13.3—Directions for Caregiver Robin (the instructor)

- *When you pretend you are washing Mrs. Baker's face, arm, and underarms, don't give any explanation.*
- *Move quickly like you are in a hurry.*
- *Respond to complaints of cold by saying "We'll be done soon."*
- *Talk with the second caregiver about your plans for this evening.*
- *Act a little annoyed that she interrupted your conversation.*
- *Don't look at her when you respond. When you do look at her, appear frustrated/not happy.*

- *After responding to her complaints of cold several times, say in an angry, loud voice, "I told you we are almost done and will be getting your clothes soon."*
- *If she raises her hand to you, say "Don't you dare! We will be done soon."*
- *Continue talking to the other caregiver. You could talk about a movie you saw over the weekend.*

Instructor:

- *Watch what happens. Pay particular attention to what I, as Caregiver Robin, do, what I say, my tone of voice and attitude. Write these things on your handout in the left column.*
- Continue the role-play until you have done all of the above.
- *What do you think Mrs. Baker felt? What behaviors did Mrs. Baker exhibit that suggested she was distressed?*
- *What did Caregiver Robin do or say that might have contributed to these feelings?*

  - Spoke harshly
  - Was disrespectful
  - Moved fast
  - Looked annoyed
  - Talked with the other caregiver and ignored care recipient
  - Focused only on getting Mrs. Baker clean, not her distressed behaviors.

- *What did Caregiver Robin NOT do?*

  - Didn't explain what she was doing
  - Didn't respond to every complaint of cold
  - Didn't smile
  - Didn't focus on Mrs. Baker as a person.

- *Will hurrying help a person feel warm rather than cold?*
- *If Caregiver Robin was to focus on Mrs. Baker while assisting her with her bath, how could she act differently? Write these on your handout.*

Instructor:

- Lead a discussion. Encourage participants to suggest behaviors that are the opposite of those listed above. Include the importance of collecting as much information as possible about Mrs. Baker so that the caregiver actions can be specific to her and her needs.

Wrap-up

- *What type of caregiver behaviors can trigger care recipient-distressed behaviors?*
- *Tell me how you will use something we discussed today with the persons for whom you care?*

Exercise 13.4—In-Room Bathing

Materials needed:

- Blackboard
- Whiteboard
- Pad on an easel or something to write down ideas and questions

Equipment for an in-bed covered massage bed bath (enough so every pair of participants can make up a kit): one large plastic bag containing:

- One large, lightweight towel
- One standard bath towel
- Two or more washcloths
- Large bath blankets.

Other supplies needed:

- No-rinse soap
- Plastic pitcher
- Rollaway bed.

Overheads:

- Consider a bed bath
- Steps in the covered massage bed bath
- Individualizing the covered massage bed bath.

Handouts:

- The covered massage bath (Table 5.17)
- Individualizing the covered massage bath (Table 5.18)
- Myths of bathing.

Learning objectives:

- To understand the benefits of in-room bathing
- To determine those persons who are appropriate for in-room bathing
- To acquire skill in one type of in-room bathing: the covered massage bed bath
- To be able to alter the covered massage bed bath in order to meet individual needs.

Outline:

- Warm-up
- Discussion of some of the myths of bathing
- Reasons for using an in-room bathing method
- Demonstration of covered massage bed bath
- Opportunity to practice covered massage bed bath
- Discussion of methods of individualizing the covered massage bed bath
- Discussion of pros and cons of the covered massage bed bath.

Examples for instructors:

1. Warm-up: Open the session with one of these exercises to create a comfortable learning environment and to encourage interaction among participants and interest in the topic.

   - Ask participants to settle back and think about a bath or shower they particularly enjoyed. Ask them to picture being in the same bath or shower—to feel the water, smell the aromas, relive the experience in their minds. Give participants a few minutes to visualize this bath and then ask them to share with the others what made that bath enjoyable. List on the board all the factors that participants mention (e.g., warm, soothing, refreshing, relaxing, invigorating). Then ask them about bathing a person with dementia. How would they describe a typical bath or shower for this person (e.g., frightening, painful, cold)?
   - Ask participants about their preferences for bathing. Use questions such as: When do you like to bathe—morning, evening, both? Do you prefer a shower? A tub bath? What do you do if you don't feel like a bath or shower but know you have areas that need cleaning?

2. Discuss some of the myths of bathing (pass out handout). Specific ones to include are:

- It takes lots of water to rinse someone.
- Families will insist on a shower or bath.

Encourage discussion of alternative methods of getting clean. Ask for suggestions and write the responses on whatever you use to write down suggestions and comments. Conclude with the statement that sometimes an in-room bath in the bed is the best choice.

3. Discuss the persons who are most likely to benefit from in-room bathing and why. These include (see overhead) those who:

- are frail and who fatigue easily
- are nonambulatory
- experience pain on transfer
- are fearful of lifts
- have acute illness
- are afraid of the shower spray
- are overstimulated in the shower
- are expressing the desire for it.

4. Demonstrate the covered massage bed bath (use overhead with steps). Give out handout with covered massage bed bath instructions.

5. Ask participants to pair up and prepare the covered massage bed bath. Have them mix the no-rinse soap, pour it into the bag with the towel and washcloths, and feel the degree of wetness. At this point you can ask for a volunteer who is willing to put on a gown and receive a modified covered massage bed bath. The person receiving the covered massage bed bath can then give feedback to the person giving it. Ask for what feels good; what doesn't feel good. An alternative to this is to have participants practice on each other using a dry towel.

6. Case study: Use a case study to help participants understand the need to individualize the covered massage bed bath just as you would any bath (use the overhead on individualizing the covered massage bed bath to stimulate discussion).

Discussion questions:

- What concerns do you have about using this as the primary method of bathing?
- What would need to be in place for you to implement this in-bed bathing method?

- How could you discuss switching from shower to in-bed bathing with the family? What points would you want to make? What possible concerns would you want to anticipate? How could you reassure them that good care will continue?

Follow-up:

The next step would be to ask for volunteers to try the covered massage bed bath with bedside consultation by the instructor. This will be an excellent opportunity to refine skills in giving the bed bath as well as to assess needs and vary the approach.

Exercise 13.5—The Learning Circle

Purpose: The learning circle is an excellent teaching tool that can be used to build trust as well as to give staff and residents a voice in decisions and solutions to problems. When staff members are involved in problem solving they often find creative ways to accomplish tasks. The learning circle also promotes relationships between employees of all levels and residents. These relationships support person-directed care and help move a facility toward culture change (see chapter 12, "Bathing as a Vehicle for Change").

Instructor Preparation:

- Work with management and nursing staff to select staff participants. Invite residents who want to be part of the discussion to attend. The ideal number of participants is 10 to 15. If the facilitator believes the discussion will provoke strong feelings of sadness, depression, grief, or anger, it is helpful to limit the number to 5 to 10.
- Arrange for a room with enough comfortable chairs for the number of participants and a quiet environment so all will be able to hear and participate.
- Choose the topic to be discussed (see suggestions that follow).

Procedure:

1. Participants sit in a circle without tables or other obstructions blocking their view of one another. Participants can include any combination of workers, residents, families, and other community members.

2. The ideal number of participants is 10 to 15. If the facilitator believes the discussion will provoke strong feelings of sadness, depression, grief, or anger, it is helpful to limit the number to 5 to 10.

3. One person is chosen to be the facilitator. The facilitator poses the question or topic to the participants, gives encouragement, and keeps the circle moving in an orderly fashion.

4. The process begins when the facilitator poses the question or issue.

5. A volunteer in the circle responds with his/her thoughts about the topic.

6. The person sitting to the right or left of the first respondent speaks next, followed one by one around the circle until everyone has spoken on the subject without interruption.

7. Participants may choose to pass rather than to speak. After everyone else in the circle has taken a turn, the facilitator goes back to those who passed and allows each of them another opportunity to respond.

8. Only after everyone has had a chance to speak is the floor opened for general discussion.

Topics or questions can be initially asked in separate groups for staff and for residents so that each feels free to speak openly. As the process moves forward, it is useful to have combined groups so each hears the thoughts and feelings of others. Here are some suggested topics or questions:

For staff

- How do you feel about how residents are currently bathed?
- What is your experience when you have to bathe a reluctant or resistive resident?
- How do you think it could be different?
- Now that you have seen the video ("Bathing Without a Battle"), do you have any thoughts on how it could be different?
- Now that we have decided we would like to make bathing more pleasant, who do you think needs to be involved in planning the change?

For residents

- What is your experience when you are showered or when you get a tub bath?
- How much choice do you feel you have in how, when, or where you are bathed?
- Do you have any thoughts on what could be done to make it more pleasant?

For combined groups:

- Now that we have decided we want to make bathing more pleasant, what ideas do you have for how we could work together to make that happen?

Exercise 13.1—Empathy

Directions for Care Receivers and Caregivers

Instructions—Care Recipients

– Remain seated

– You can't talk

– Put your hands behind your back

– Try to do what you are told to do

– Close your eyes now and keep them closed

Instructions—Caregiver

– Take the wipe out of the baggie

– Mumble, *"Need to get this done. Hurry up!"*

– Touch your partner on the neck with the wipe

– Tug at his/her clothes

– Wipe his/her arm

Exercise 13.2—Physical and Emotional Triggers of Behaviors Script/Directions

----

Scene 13.2A—Script

Caregiver: "Hi, Mrs. Peters, it is time for your bath. Let's go to the bathroom."

Mrs. Peters: "No, I have already had my bath."

Caregiver: "You have not had your bath yet, Mrs. Peters. Come on, it won't take long."

Mrs. Peters (say a little louder): "I told you I had a bath!"

Caregiver: "Mrs. Peters, you are dirty. Don't you want to get nice and clean?"

Mrs. Peters: "I am not dirty!!! I already had a bath and I am NOT going to take a second one!! Leave me alone!" (shake your fist at the caregiver)

Scene 13.2B—Directions

Caregiver: Pretend you are washing Mrs. Peters's arm, lifting it to wash her underarm.

Scene 13.2C—Directions

Caregiver: Continue to pretend to wash Mrs. Peters.

Exercise 13.3—Caregiver Behaviors as Triggers

Directions for Care Receiver and Second Caregiver

Mrs. Baker, the Care Receiver

– Every few seconds say "I'm cold!," "I already had a bath."

– No matter what Caregiver Robin says, repeat "I'm cold."

– When Caregiver Robin tries to lift your arm, pull it back, saying "No, no, no!" and raise your hand and say "I'm going to hit you!"

Second Caregiver

You will be helping Caregiver Robin give Mrs. Baker a shower by just holding her arm.

Caregiver Robin will be talking to you. Just appear to be interested by nodding your head and saying "uh huh."

Exercise 13.3　Caregiver Behavior as Triggers

What did Caregiver Robin do?	What should Caregiver Robin have done?
What Caregiver Robin did not do	

BATHING WITHOUT A BATTLE: COMMON MYTHS RELATED TO BATHING

- **It takes lots of water to get people clean.**
  In health care and home settings, people have kept clean without the benefit of showers, tubs, or running water. Careful washing, with attention to details, is more important than how much water you use.

- **If caregivers are delaying, deferring, shortening, or adapting the bath or shower, they are trying to get out of work.**
  This may be necessary to create a person-directed plan that meets the person's special needs. They are still responsible for maintaining the person's hygiene but need freedom to adjust the method.

- **Families will insist on a shower or tub bath.**
  Families, like the rest of us, need to be educated. If they are presented with the problem (the person dislikes or fights the bath or shower) and alternative suggestions, usually they understand and are agreeable to a trial of other methods.

- **There will be more infections and skin problems.**
  Many people have not gotten into a shower or tub for years, yet they are clean and have no increased infections or skin problems.

- **People always feel better after they have a bath or shower.**
  If it is forced, people feel attacked, demoralized, fearful, and it is an exhausting process.

- **You have to just go ahead because for most people who resist, there won't be a "good" time.**
  For most people with dementia, it is possible to develop a plan that keeps them clean and avoids the battle by adapting the approach, method, day, and time of day.

- **They just forget about the battle so it doesn't matter.**
  Many people who are forced to bathe stay upset for hours.

- **Regulators, advocates, and families will see it as possible neglect.**
  When you are rethinking what is currently accepted practice, be proactive and educate all players. Let people know what you are doing and why. Frame it as a better way of meeting someone's needs.

- **The person-directed approach will take more time, and we don't have it.**
  For most people, if you are organized, have your supplies handy, and are familiar with the techniques, it can be done in the same amount of time. If overall you end up bathing some people less frequently, then there may be a decrease in time spent bathing.

OVERHEAD / PowerPoint slide

Bed Bath

Consider a bed bath for persons who:

- are frail (who fatigue easily)
- are nonambulatory
- experience pain on transfer
- are fearful of lifts
- experience acute illness
- are afraid of the shower spray
- are overstimulated in the shower
- express a desire for it.

Covered Massage Bed Bath

- Prepare the person.
- Prepare the bath.
- Bathe the person.
- Allow person to rest.

OVERHEAD / PowerPoint slide

Table Individualizing the Covered Massage Bed Bath

Concern	Action
Cold	<ul><li>Cover with dry towel</li><li>Double bag wet towel</li><li>Remove wet towel quickly</li></ul>
Pain when turning over	<ul><li>Wash back, rectum, and genitals while standing</li></ul>
Agitation	<ul><li>Have one person talk while a second one washes</li><li>Use other distracters</li><li>Keep lights low</li><li>Play soft music</li></ul>

Case Example

Mr. Nash is a 75-year-old man who is severely demented. He is incontinent of bowel and bladder and can speak very few words. He yells every time you try to move him. He cries throughout his shower and is difficult to console. He seems to be sensitive to cold as he keeps trying to cover himself. His daughter visits every day and is concerned about his health and well-being.

Case Example

Mrs. Pearl is a very active woman in the middle stage of Alzheimer's disease. She wanders the halls during the day, greets people with a smile, and then moves on. She enjoys dancing and loves "big band" music. She is very agitated during the shower. She keeps trying to get out of the chair and leave the bathroom. Her rectum is very sensitive due to hemorrhoids, and she yells and squirms when it is being washed.

CHAPTER 14

Taking Care of Yourself: Strategies for Caregivers

Joyce H. Rasin

THE STRESSES OF CAREGIVING

As a caregiver, you spend many hours a day attending to other people. But how much time do you actually spend caring for yourself? Caring for yourself is important, too, because if you don't take care of yourself, pretty soon you won't be able to do your best for others. Caregiving can be rewarding and challenging. However, providing care to persons with dementia who have behavioral symptoms can be stressful. Stress occurs when you experience the daily events in your life as potentially harmful (e.g., leading to loss) or when you see the challenges in your life as difficult, painful, or unfair. Stress also occurs when you are concerned that you may not have the resources to cope with these events or the daily "hassles" of caregiving. Stressors in your life can be personal, interpersonal, or environmental. Examples of typical daily stressors for a paid caregiver include:

- Mr. H. continually begs you not to give him a shower. It makes you feel really bad to do it anyway, but it has to be done because it is his bath day.
- When you try to wash Ms. P's hair she pushes your hand away and calls you a name.
- Mr. M. starts to cry when you tell him he can't go home.
- Ms. R. moans whenever you move her leg.
- Your schedule changes with little notice.
- You have a disagreement with a supervisor or coworker.
- The shower room is too hot.
- There are not enough towels or washcloths to do the job well.

Typical daily stressors for family caregivers include:

- Your husband doesn't recognize you when you come to assist him with bathing.
- Your mother is up all night wandering in the house, and you are fearful she will get out and get lost.
- Your wife is no longer safe in the kitchen and you don't know how to cook or use the appliances.
- You have to cut through the red tape of health insurance carriers.
- You are having trouble finding a sitter so you can go to the doctor.

Recognizing those situations you find stressful is the first step in dealing with them. If the stress you experience from caregiving is not minimized or reduced, your physical, emotional, and/or social health may be affected. Once you recognize the source of your stress, you can begin to find ways to manage your reaction to it.

Personal Stress Responses

Sometimes as a caregiver you are so focused on the care recipient that you don't notice your own feelings. Throughout your day you have moments when you feel stressed and moments when you feel relaxed. Try to become aware of the first sign of stress so it won't increase. Think about your typical day. To identify some of the ways that you respond to stressors, complete "Personal Reaction to Stress" in Exhibit 14.1.

You can respond to stress with your body (physically), through your feelings (emotionally), or in your thinking

EXHIBIT 14.1   Personal Reaction to Stress

When you're feeling stressed and anxious, what do you typically experience? Check all that apply.

1. My heart beats faster.
2. I get diarrhea.
3. I have sweaty palms.
4. I lose my appetite.
5. I feel anxious.
6. I become very critical of other people.
7. I tend to cry.
8. I withdraw from my family and friends.
9. I become forgetful.
10. I lose my concentration easily.
11. I can't get as much done as usual.
12. I lose interest.

(cognitively). Any of these responses is normal and is your body's way of letting you know, consciously or unconsciously, that something is a stressor. In the "Personal Reaction to Stress" checklist, physical responses are Nos. 1, 2, 3, and 4; emotional responses are Nos. 5, 6, 7, and 8; and cognitive responses are Nos. 9, 10, 11, and 12. You may have more responses that are physical, whereas another person will have more emotional responses. It is also possible to have responses from all categories. The type and the number of your responses will differ from other people's responses. Being aware of your reactions can help you develop ways to care for yourself.

Burnout

All caregivers are at risk of burnout. You may be on the verge of burning out when the stressors you experience from caregiving overpower your ability to cope with them. Burnout may result from chronic stressful situations also. The classic symptoms of burnout are loss of energy and enthusiasm, increased dissatisfaction, pessimism, and inefficiency. You may feel overloaded or as if you don't know what you are doing anymore. Burnout increases your risk for developing physical problems such as high blood pressure and heart disease or emotional problems such as depression. Burnout begins slowly and increases gradually, so catching it early is important. See Table 14.1 for some warning signs that a stressful situation is overwhelming your ability to cope with it and that you are burning out.

If one or more of the previously mentioned signs occurs frequently, you are a candidate for burnout. Turn to a close friend or confidant or ask your primary health care provider or spiritual advisor for assistance in coping with your stressors. Many people try to relieve their stress by smoking, excessive drinking, overeating, or taking unnecessary pills. These actions also can have a negative impact on your health. Instead make a health care plan for yourself. Incorporate into your lifestyle some alternative healthier strategies for coping with stress. The next section of the chapter outlines some healthy coping approaches.

Startegies for Self-Care

Develop a plan for self-care to prevent or diminish stress in your life. Some strategies are appropriate for all care providers, whereas others are specific to either paid or family caregivers. You may find some of the following strategies helpful for your self-care plan.

Strategies for All Care Providers

Physical Health

Staying physically healthy will help you stay emotionally healthy. Your health is one of the most important

TABLE 14.1   Signs of Burnout

How often do these occur?	Never	Sometimes	Frequently
1. Coming down with more colds and headaches than usual.	☐	☐	☐
2. Can't get excited about your job.	☐	☐	☐
3. Don't enjoy giving care to care recipient.	☐	☐	☐
4. Lie awake at night worrying.	☐	☐	☐
5. Suddenly losing weight without trying.	☐	☐	☐
6. Frequent conflicts with care recipient, coworkers, and/or family.	☐	☐	☐
7. Cry every day.	☐	☐	☐
8. Resent suggestions from coworkers and family for doing things.	☐	☐	☐
9. Feeling tired all day.	☐	☐	☐

resources you have and is essential if you want to be a long-term caregiver. So there are two reasons to maintain your health—for your own well-being and for the well-being of the person(s) for whom you care. Diet, exercise, and sleep will improve your ability to cope with the stress you experience from caregiving.

A *balanced diet* is important for good health. Every day you should have:

- grains
- fruits and vegetables
- milk, cheese, or yogurt
- poultry, fish, meat, eggs, or dried beans
- 2 quarts of water
- sugar, in moderation
- no more than one alcoholic drink
- low fat and cholesterol.

Choose foods in each category that you like. Take time to relax as you eat. Try not to read or watch television while eating so you can be aware of the flavors. Food is a necessity and a pleasure, so enjoy!

Regular exercise. Pick an activity that you enjoy. Three types of exercises are important for physical fitness:

- Endurance or aerobic
- Strengthening or muscle building
- Flexibility.

Endurance/aerobic exercises increase your heart and lung function and should be done at least three times per week. Walking, swimming, biking, and dancing are all aerobic exercises. Start slowly and increase the intensity gradually. Even a 5-minute walk a day is a good start. If you can't talk while you are exercising, you are going too fast. See your physician or other primary health care provider before you begin your routine if you have heart trouble, chest pain, diabetes, high blood pressure, dizziness, or arthritis. To complete your fitness program, include exercises to strengthen your muscles (lifting weights such as hand weights, soup cans, or water bottles) and to stretch your muscles. The National Institute on Aging puts out an excellent exercise guide that is available for free and a videotape for a small fee (see Resources at the end of this chapter). Many video stores and libraries also have exercise videos or DVDs.

Sleep. Getting an adequate number of hours of sleep is very important. The long-term effects of sleep loss increase the risk for many chronic diseases such as hyper-

tension, depression, and stroke (Institute of Medicine, 2006). Sleep is a time for your mind and your body to rest. Having good sleep habits (regular bedtime and comfortable room environment) will help you rest. Try not to read or watch television in bed so that going to bed is associated with going to sleep.

Learning to Relax

Learning to physically and mentally relax is an important skill to develop. Two ways to relax are "attending to simple pleasures" and "achieving the relaxation response."

Attend to the simple pleasures in your life. Simple pleasures are activities that bring a smile to your face and a feeling of contentment. They are not expensive nor do they take time to plan. They allow you to appreciate what is happening to you in the moment and not to worry about the past or the future. Some examples of simple pleasures are:

- Walking through a wooded area in the fall where all you can hear is the crunching of leaves from the pressure of your footsteps.
- Filling the tub full of warm water, adding your favorite bubble bath or bath oil, soft music in the background, a burning candle, and a pillow for your neck and head. (Spend about 20 minutes of solitude in your bath.)
- Sharing a funny story with a friend.

Identify some simple pleasures for yourself and build them into your daily routine. Enjoy them throughout the day.

Caregiver Wisdom

It's important to focus on the person, but if I'm distracted by worries, I stop for a minute, talk to myself, and then refocus.

Rosa Stephens, CNA, Oxford Manor, Oxford, NC

The relaxation response is a physical state of rest that alters the physical and emotional response to stress. For over 35 years, Dr. Herbert Benson and colleagues (2007) have been teaching persons how to elicit this response as part of a program to decrease stress-related medical disorders. If the body can relax, the mind will follow. Just

EXHIBIT 14.2   The Relaxation Response

- Select your focus word(s)—a word with special meaning for you.
- Sit quietly in a comfortable position.
- Close your eyes.
- Let your muscles go limp, stretch to let go of any tension.
- Breathe slowly and naturally. Repeat your focus words as you exhale.
- When other thoughts come into your head, just ignore them and return to your focus word(s).
- Continue for 10–20 minutes each time.

When you are finished, don't stand immediately but sit quietly for a minute and let your everyday thoughts return.

---

two things must be completed: (a) a focus word, phrase, or prayer must be selected, such as "Peace," "Calm," "Relax," "Om," "The Lord is my shepherd"; and (b) everyday thoughts that come to mind must be disregarded. See Exhibit 14.2 for steps to achieve the relaxation response.

Support Network

Throughout this book the importance of the caregiving relationship has been emphasized. Supportive relationships help minimize the effects of all types of stressors, including those associated with providing care. Find a person or persons in whom you can confide or with whom you feel comfortable talking. Confidants can be found among your coworkers, family members, or friends. These individuals not only provide emotional support, they also help you learn new problem-solving skills.

Attitudes and Beliefs

Positive self-talk. Your thoughts influence your feelings. In other words, what you tell yourself is what you will feel. If you are involved in negative self-talk, you are encouraging yourself to feel negative. Use positive self-talk to prepare yourself for using positive self-talk; write down some positive statements about yourself. For example, "I did a really good job getting Mr. M. to change his clothes." "I am capable of giving excellent care." When you are feeling anxious and not good about yourself, take out your positive self-talk statements and read them.

Caregiver Wisdom

I try to keep a positive outlook. I make a list of all the good memories, and when I get down, I read that list to remind me of the good things. I depend a lot on my church and spiritual beliefs to give me support. I attend Bible study classes. I garden. Those are all therapeutic for me.

Pat Ehresman, in-home caregiver for her mother, who has Parkinson's disease, and her husband, who has dementia

---

Professional Counseling and Therapy

If you have tried everything suggested here and still feel physically or emotionally exhausted, you may benefit from professional assistance to help you identify positive steps to manage your stress. Some people you could contact if you decide you need help include:

- priest, pastor, or rabbi
- your physician or primary care provider
- Clinical psychologist, psychiatric mental health nurse specialist, or social worker. Many of these health professionals can be found at a local mental health clinic.

Strategies Specifically for Paid Caregivers

As paid caregivers, your situation is a little different from that of family caregivers. The long-term care of several persons who may have mental and/or physical impairments can be very stressful. Also, coworkers and supervisors may contribute to your stress, or help relieve it, so relationships with others are especially important. Adding a stressful work situation to everyday life may make coping more difficult. Consider the following in addition to the strategies already discussed in this chapter.

- *Support at work.* Support at work can be informal or organized. Talking with a coworker from another unit or floor who isn't involved in your immediate caregiving situation can provide you with a nonjudgmental listener. By talking through the situation, you may view it in a different way. Support can be supplied more formally through team meetings, team venting sessions, or your clinical supervisor in a positive work environment. Having colleagues who not only listen to your frustrations but also provide feedback and help with problem solving can be very beneficial.

- *Change.* You may have talked with coworkers and clinical managers/supervisors about a difficult situation with a care recipient. You may have brainstormed about different ways to resolve the situation and tried alternative approaches. However, sometimes because of other stressors occurring in your life, you are not as resilient and may need some respite. Talk with your clinical supervisor about a short-term change in assignment.
- *Relax.* Yes, it is possible to relax at work. On your break, if the weather allows, go outside for a few minutes and enjoy the sun, the wind, or even the rain. Forget about what else you have to do and be aware of your surroundings. Give your body and your mind a chance to slow down. Pause, breathe deeply a few times, smile, and let your body relax.

Caregiver Wisdom

When stressed at work, we would talk among ourselves and try to work it out. We tried to support each other. I also found the nurses and doctors helpful. I could talk to them about personal or work-related issues.
Tom Pruitt, HCT, retired from John Umstead Hospital, Butner, NC

Strategies Specifically for Family Caregivers

- *Be realistic about what is possible.* There is a limit to what any one person can do in one day. First, you have to differentiate between needs and wants. Although you may have a list of things you want done, all of them may not need to be done. Needs and wants will differ by family, and only you can make the choice. What you value most is what is important, not what others think. Even after you identify your needs, you still may have to set limits on what you can do within a day. Be realistic and don't be afraid to ask for assistance.
- *Get help from your family and friends.* How often has someone told you to "let me know when I can help you"? Many times other people want to help, but they don't know how they can be of assistance.

They need some direction. Make a list of what needs to be done. Perhaps you need someone to sit with your family member while you do errands or so that you can focus on an activity within your home without an interruption. Make sure some of the activities on the list are for your self-care. Taking a walk, going to the movies, or taking a nap. Asking for help is actually a strength, not a weakness. You can't do it alone.
- *Share your feelings with others.* Sharing feelings with a close friend or family member helps get them out in the open and lessens the impact of negative emotions. Pick someone with whom you can confide or comfortably talk to without censoring your feelings. Many caregivers also have gained strength through support from different organizations such as the Alzheimer's Association, American Heart Association, and American Cancer Society. Check the newspaper for meeting listings. Caregivers who belong to a faith community may find that the spiritual leader (priest, pastor, rabbi) can provide guidance.

Caregiver Wisdom

I accept my new limitations. I recognize that I don't have the same level of freedom that I had before. I can't just go off shopping or visiting with friends. I have to plan ahead for those things to happen now, and it is helpful that I have come to accept that this is true and that I have to ask for help to get away when I need to. I have also come to accept the new limitations of my mother and husband. I have dropped all expectations about how they were or should be and recognize that they have changed and I need to adjust. It makes life easier.
Pat Ehresman, in-home caregiver for her mother, who has Parkinson's disease, and her husband, who has dementia

Gender Differences

Traditionally, most family caregivers have been women. However, as the population ages and people live longer, more men are finding themselves in caregiving roles by choice or by circumstance. Men may have some different issues. They have lost their key source of emotional support if the care recipient is their spouse. In addition, because traditionally they have not been responsible for

TABLE 14.2 Self-Care Strategies

Directions: Read each statement. How often do they occur now?	Never	Sometimes	Frequently
1. I eat at least one hot, balanced meal a day.	☐	☐	☐
2. I get 7 to 8 hours of sleep a night.	☐	☐	☐
3. I give and receive affection regularly.	☐	☐	☐
4. I exercise at least three times a week.	☐	☐	☐
5. I take fewer than five alcoholic drinks a week.	☐	☐	☐
6. I am the appropriate weight for my height.	☐	☐	☐
7. I get strength from my spiritual beliefs.	☐	☐	☐
8. I am regularly involved in a social activity.	☐	☐	☐
9. I have a network of friends and acquaintances.	☐	☐	☐
10. I have one or more friends to confide in about personal matters.	☐	☐	☐
11. I am able to speak openly about my feelings when I am angry or worried.	☐	☐	☐
12. I do something for fun on a regular basis.	☐	☐	☐
13. I am able to organize my time effectively.	☐	☐	☐
14. I take quiet time for myself during the day.	☐	☐	☐
TOTAL	☐	☐	☐

Count the number of "Frequently" responses. How many do you have?
What can you do to change "Never" to "Frequently"?
Choose three strategies from this chapter to use as part of your self-care plan.

the day-to-day homemaking chores, they may be at a loss. Men may benefit from a support group for men only and community resources for meals, personal care, housecleaning, and shopping. The local Area Agency on Aging provides information and referral services. See "Eldercare Locator" on the resource list.

SUMMARY

Being a sensitive caregiver has the potential to be stressful. If you find that you are experiencing stress from the caregiving, develop a plan for self-care. Without a plan for self-care, you may become overwhelmed or burned out, which could result in physical and emotional problems. Several strategies have been described that can either decrease your vulnerability to stress or help you manage and cope with stressful situations. Evaluate your use of self-care strategies by answering the questions in Table 14.2.

Then, list three strategies that you can include in your plan for self-care.

Strategies Selected for My Self-Care

1.
2.
3.

See the resources at the end of this chapter for sources of additional information. Remember, you need to take care of yourself if you are going to care for others over the long haul. Finding meaning and pleasure in caregiving will be your reward.

REFERENCES

Benson-Henry Institute for Mind Body Medicine, Massachusetts General Hospital. (2007). Retrieved May 6, 2007, from http://www.mbmi.org/programs/default.asp

Institute of Medicine. (2006). Sleep disorders and sleep deprivation: An unmet public health problem. Retrieved May 6, 2007, from http://www.iom.edu/CMS/3740/23160/33668.aspx

APPENDIX

Resources

Addresses, telephone numbers, and/or Web site locations are provided. As long as you use sites developed by reputable organizations and agencies, they are a good source of current, reliable, and free information. If you don't have access to the Internet, many local public libraries have it. Ask your librarian to help you locate the Web page.

Alzheimer's Association
70 E. Lake Street, Suite 600
Chicago, IL 60601
1-800-621-0379
An "Educational Center" is available with information to assist in learning caregiving skills. There is also an interactive tool to help family caregivers find qualified caregivers.
http://www.alz.org

Alzheimer's Disease Education and Referral Center
1-800-438-4380
An information specialist can help you obtain information about dementia and related services. The Web site provides comprehensive information about Alzheimer's disease, and resources are available from the National Institute on Aging (e.g., clinical trials, publications, e-mail alerts).
http://www.nia.nih.gov/alzheimers

Alzheimer's Foundation of America
Provides care and services to individuals confronting dementia and Alzheimer's disease, caregivers, and families through member organizations. Sponsors programs and has a free newsletter.
www.alzfdn.org

American Association for Retired Persons (AARP)
AARP has a section on its Web site for "Caregiving." Articles are provided to help family caregivers care for themselves and for the physical, psychological, social, and financial needs of their family member.
http://www.aarp.org/families/caregiving/

American Heart Association online "Fitness Center" includes information about evaluating fitness, an exercise diary, and fitness resources.
www.justmove.org

American Stroke Association
Extensive information for family caregivers on a Web site called "Heart of Caregiving." You can sign up for a monthly e-newsletter that is said to provide tips and resources for caregivers.
http://www.strokeassociation.org/presenter.jhtml? identifier=3042552

County or city:
Social services department or mental health department (Check telephone book for local listings.)

Eldercare locator
Can direct at no charge to the nearest Area Agency on Aging that knows local resources such as housekeeping, personal care services, or Meals on Wheels. You can use the following Web site or talk with an information specialist at 1-800-677-1116. Spanish-speaking specialists are available. This is a service of the U.S. Administration on Aging.
http://www.eldercare.gov/Eldercare/Public/Home.asp

Food and Nutrition Information—MyPyramid
On this Web site you can obtain a personalized eating plan based on the latest dietary guidelines when you enter your age, height, weight, and sex. You can also assess your daily intake by entering the food you have eaten in one day. The Web site will compare your information to the recommended guidelines. You can track what you eat for a year. This Web site was developed by the Center for Nutrition Policy and Promotion, U.S. Department of Agriculture.
http://www.mypyramid.gov/

National Alliance for Caregiving
4720 Montgomery Lane Suite 642
Bethesda, MD 20814
This Web site provides access to a broad spectrum of resources including (a) tips and guides, including Family Caregiving 101—information to help with day-to-day challenges; and (b) Family Care Resource Connection publications and reports.
http://www.caregiving.org

National Family Caregiver Support Program Resource Room
Sponsored by the U.S. Administration on Aging. This Web site contains information for family and paid caregivers.
http://www.aoa.gov/prof/aoaprog/caregiver/caregiver. asp

National Institute on Aging
Has exercise video of stretching, balance, and strength training exercises in either VHS or DVD format for $7. A free exercise guide is also available. Can order online or from the following address:

NIAIC, Dept. W
P.O. Box 8057
Gaithersburg, MD 20898-8057
1-800-222-2225
http://www.niapublications.org/exercisevideo/
exercisevhs.asp

National Family Caregivers Association (NFCA)—
Provides information and tips for caregivers. It also includes a special section about caring for persons with
specific conditions or diseases, such as Alzheimer's disease. Caregivers can also connect with other caregivers
by using the message boards on the Web site or by attending NFCA conferences.
NFCA
10400 Connecticut Avenue, Suite 500
Kensington, MD 20895-3944
Toll Free: 1-800-896-3650
Phone: 301-942-6430
Fax: 301-942-2302
http://www.nfcacares.org/
General e-mail: info@thefamilycaregiver.org

Mental Health America (formerly National Mental
Health Association)
2000 N. Beauregard Street, 6th Floor, Alexandria, VA
22311
Phone: 703-684-7722
Fax: 703-684-5968
Toll free: 1-800-969-6642
TTY Line: 1-800-433-5959
Provides information about mental health issues.
http://www.nmha.org

Pillemer, Karl. *The Nursing Assistant's Survival Guide.*
Written for nursing assistants to help deal with the stres-
sors that can lead to burnout. For additional information
and order information, see the publisher's Web site:
http://www.frontlinepub.com/fln_nursesur.html
Telephone: 1-888-427-5800
Fax: 1-518-881-1266
E-mail: tl.frontline@thomson.com

APPENDIX A

Measuring Success: A Quality Improvement Program for Person-Directed Bathing

Anytime you are trying to change practice, it is useful and necessary to determine a practical, valid, and reliable way to measure effectiveness. A formal complex study is not necessary, but some way of monitoring success is. Here are some suggested ways that this could be done with bathing as a quality improvement program. In this model, each person acts as his/her own control and data is collected before and after an intervention. A direct caregiver working with a supervisor or educator will do most of the work. This two-person team will meet regularly, review progress, generate new ideas, and test them out. A program like this addresses OBRA-87 guidelines for nursing home settings and is often favorably received by state surveyors. Plus your staff members will improve in their ability to solve care problems.

FOCUS ON THE PERSON BEING BATHED

1. **Select the person(s) for whom you wish to create a person-directed bathing approach.**

   As mentioned in Chapter 12, it may be useful to start with one or two people in one section of the facility and expand later. It is also helpful to start with less complicated behaviors and persons. Choose a person with strengths you can use such as the ability to understand what you say. Don't pick your most challenging resident. Wait until you have gained some experience.

2. **Select the caregiver(s) who will be working with each person being bathed.**

   Select one caregiver to work with each person being bathed. If two or more caregivers are needed, it is helpful to have a consistent second person. This is not crucial as long as the primary person is the same and guides the interaction. This primary person should be someone who is interested in learning new methods for making bathing pleasurable.

3. **Decide what target behaviors you wish to alter for each person and set measurable goals.**

   These can be positive behaviors you wish to increase or negative behaviors you wish to decrease (Table 5.1). You are identifying how you will know if your approaches are successful; in other words, what you want to change.

4. **Decide on an observational method to measure change.**

   Here are some suggested ways to measure change in the behaviors of the person being bathed:

   a. *Direct observation:* Have an uninvolved staff person present when the person is being bathed. Choose this person carefully, as he/she will need to be objective and unbiased. Develop a form that lists your target behaviors and ask the person to count them during the bath. The Behavior Checklist (Appendix B) could be used for this.

b. *Recalling and recording:* After the bath ask the bathing caregiver(s) to recall target behaviors and record them on a form. The Behavior Checklist (Appendix B) could be used for this.

c. *Videotaping:* As mentioned earlier, videotaping the bath can be a useful learning tool. It can also be used as a method of measuring outcomes. Obtain written permission from the family and verbal assent from the person before each bath. Tape three baseline (pretest) and three postintervention (posttest baths). Then ask a staff member (who is actively involved in the resident's care) to view the tapes without knowledge of which tape was pre and which was post. This is a stronger methodology for evaluation because it eliminates some potential bias. The Behavior Checklist (Appendix B) could be used to count resident behaviors. Great caution must be used to ensure the confidentiality of the tapes and who views them. They must be destroyed when the evaluation is complete.

Each method has pros and cons. The direct observation requires an extra person. The recall method relies on the memory of an involved and, therefore, potentially biased participant. The videotaping may be seen as too intrusive and time consuming.

5. **Decide on any physiologic measures you wish to monitor.**

Identify the physical concerns (odor, overall appearance, skin problems, etc) you have related to changing the bathing program for the person. Develop a data collection method. These may be very simple such as a narrative note or a scale from 0–3. If you use a scale, having descriptors and definitions for each point on the scale will make it easier to use. For example, 0 could be labeled as "0" or "no odor," and 3 could be labeled as "a lot" or "very strong odor." These labels "anchor" the points on the scale and help clarify what each one means.

6. **Collect your baseline data.**

Baseline data is information collected before you try a new method or approach. Have the caregiver(s) bathe the person in the usual way (tub, shower, bed bath). Collect data using your chosen method for three baths.

7. **Decide on possible causes/triggers for behaviors.**

Following the collection of the baseline data, you will need to provide some education and training (see chapter 13) for the intervention team (the direct caregiver and the supervisor or educator.) They will then brainstorm and problem solve before the next bath. You may find the Behavior Tracking Log (Figure 4.1) and Bathing Preferences and Practices Form (Appendix, chapter 4) helpful. The baseline data will also be helpful for you to use in problem solving.

8. **Select solutions/approaches you wish to try.**

Chapter 5 will be very useful in helping you decide on new interventions for the specific problems you have identified. Check the tables that are available for problems such as pain, being cold, refusing to enter bathing room for solutions. Use the Intervention Planning Form (chapter 5, Exhibit 5.1) as a tool.

9. **Test solutions.**

With the next bath, the designated caregiver will try out the selected solutions. Following each bath or shower, those involved will debrief, brainstorm, and evaluate the selected interventions. Again, the Intervention Planning Form (chapter 5, Exhibit 5.1) will be useful. Decide what worked, what didn't work, and why and what you will try next time.

10. **Finalize your care plan.**

Continue this process for several baths or until the caregiver feels that he/she has reached the goals set for the target behaviors or has run out of ideas/solutions. The number of trials needed to finalize the care plan will vary from person to person. The average is about 3–4 times, but some persons' discomfort can be reduced in one trial. For others, some discomfort and distress may remain. Six to eight attempts to revise care approaches are probably a sufficient trial. Write up a person-directed bathing care plan that the caregiver will follow during the posttest data collection period.

11. **Collect your postintervention or posttest data.**

Using the same data collection method you used for the baseline baths, collect data on the next three baths, with the caregiver(s) using the person-directed bathing care plan developed in the intervention/solution testing process.

12. **Analyze your data.**

Look at the data you collected before the intervention and after the intervention was introduced, comparing the counts on the targeted behaviors between the two time periods. Average the scores or numbers for the behaviors and physiologic measures observed in the baseline baths and do the same for the behaviors observed in the baths completed after the intervention was introduced. Compare the pretest scores with the posttest scores. Was there an overall increase in positive behaviors and decrease in negative behaviors? Did scores on physiological measures indicate improvement? If so, the intervention was helpful. If not, it was not successful. Use the data and the insights of the team to decide what the next step should be.

13. **Share the results with other involved parties.**

Use the data to further your goal of creating a positive bathing experience for all residents and staff. Chart the results to show the outcomes. If you are in a nursing home setting, you may wish to share the study with state surveyors. Also, include this information in the resident's medical chart so that other caregivers will be aware of what worked and what didn't work and progress that has been made toward goals.

14. **Expand your program to include others who show discomfort during bathing.**

Once you have achieved success with one or two persons, talk with staff about other persons who need a person-directed bath plan. Also invite different staff to participate. Follow the steps 3–13.

FOCUS ON CAREGIVER BEHAVIORS

So far the focus on analysis and study has been on the person being bathed. As we have stated in the book, that is only half of the equation. The actions of the caregiver and the quality of the relationship are a major factor in determining the outcome. The same intervention carried out by caregivers with different styles and motivations can yield very different results.

If you wish to also evaluate the caregiver's behavior, use the direct observation or the videotape method. Using the same approach as described for the person being bathed, ask the observer to fill out the Caregiver Behavior Checklist (Appendix C) for baseline (pretest) and postintervention (posttest) baths. An unbiased observer is very important here also. For the videotaped method, the rater would watch the video a second time to rate the caregiver using the checklist. The observer may also wish to compare the observed caregiver's actions against the written care plan and make an estimate of the percentage of the care plan carried out during the bath. This method of data collection will help you gather data-based evidence to guide you in implementing and evaluating a care plan.

Behavior Rating Checklist

Name: _____ Date: _____ Time: _____ Recorder: _____

Record the frequency of each behavior by placing an x in the box beside the behavior each time it occurs. If two behaviors occur simultaneously, rate BOTH. Definitions are on the back.

Behaviors suggesting discomfort*   Behaviors indicating comfort

Frequency	Behavior
	Avoid bathing
	Biting
	Closed fist
	Complaints
	Finger pointing
	Grabbing or attempts to grab
	Hitting, pushing, scratching, punching, or attempts
	Hostile language
	Kicks or attempts to kick
	Leaving
	Spitting
	Throwing things
	Other agitated or aggressive behavior

Frequency	Behavior
	Hugging/kissing
	Smiling/laughing
	Singing
	Thanks or compliments caregiver
	Other positive behaviors (list)

*HIGHLIGHT BEHAVIORS THAT OCCURRED DURING THE BASELINE BATHS. DID THESE BEHAVIORS IMPROVE?

OVERALL ASSESSMENT OF PERSON'S DISCOMFORT

     1   2   3   4   5   6

Completely comfortable   Extremely uncomfortable

Comments: (note anything unusual or surprising that occurred)_____

_____

_____

DEFINITIONS

Avoiding bathing	resists being bathed, e.g., moves body to avoid being bathed, turns head away when face is being washed, includes avoiding being undressed. If the resident grabs the caregiver, rate as grabbing.
Biting	bites, or attempts to bite, chomps, gnaws (on caregiver only)
Closed fist	closes one or both fists
Complaints	expresses displeasure in words (e.g. "I am cold")
Finger pointing	points finger at caregiver
Grabbing	grabs or attempts to grab onto people or objects inappropriately; snatches, seizes roughly. DO NOT rate if resident is already grabbing object/person unless resident grabs object/person with other hand. Do not rate if resident is holding on for safety reasons.
Hitting, pushing, scratching	physically abuses or attempts to abuse caregiver with hand or handheld object or with other body parts (head, whole body), includes pushing, shoving, scratching (contact occurs)
Hostile language	cursing/obscene/vulgar language, verbal threats, name calling
Hugging/Kissing	resident hugs or kisses caregiver
Kicking or attempts to kick	strikes forcefully with foot or leg (contact occurs) or swings out leg and foot with force toward caregiver
Leaving	tries to get out of shower area or resists going to shower area. This is "escape" behavior. REQUIRES caregiver intervention—the caregiver may block an exit with his/her body, may take hold of the resident to keep him/her in the shower, may pull/push on the resident to get him/her to walk to the shower.
Singing	sings or hums
Spitting	spits on purpose (does not have to be at caregiver)
Other agitation or aggression	shows physical signs of distress including repetitive mannerisms, hyperactivity, wringing hands, flailing arms, nonpurposeful movement of the feet, legs, or torso
Thanks or compliments caregiver	expresses appreciation to caregiver; expresses praise and/or admiration
Throwing things	forcefully throws object, knocks object off surface

Caregiver Behavior Checklist

Name of caregiver: _____ Person being bathed: _____ Date of bath: _____

	Never	Almost Never	Occasionally	Often	Almost Always	Always
VERBAL COMMUNICATION						
Praises resident	1	2	3	4	5	6
Uses a calm voice	1	2	3	4	5	6
Speaks respectfully	1	2	3	4	5	6
Expresses concern/interest	1	2	3	4	5	6
Speaks directly to resident	1	2	3	4	5	6
TASK PRESENTATION						
Prepares resident for the task	1	2	3	4	5	6
Bathes at a pace appropriate for this resident	1	2	3	4	5	6
NONVERBAL COMMUNICATION						
Gently touches resident	1	2	3	4	5	6
Is flexible with the bathing routine	1	2	3	4	5	6
Makes eye contact with the resident	1	2	3	4	5	6
INDEPENDENCE (assess if appropriate)						
Encourages independence	1	2	3	4	5	6

TOTAL: _____

Index

Impaired judgment, 67
Impulse control, 23, 27
In-bed bathing, 54
In-bed inflatable basin method, 58
Incentives
    training, 143
Incontinence, 54, 59
Individualized ADL prescription form, 74
Individualizing the covered massage bath, 56t
Indocin, 83
Indomethacin, 83
Infection and micro-organisms prevention
    guidelines during bathing activities, 89–90
Infection control, 89
Inflatable tub, 120
In-room bathing, 151
Intervention planning form, 59–61
Intervention planning table, 35
Invitation to the bath, 5–6

Jelly-in-the-hair, 58
Judgment, 28

Keri oil, 90

Lavender bath, 81
Learning circle, 133–134, 134t, 143, 144, 152–153
Learning. *See* Training
    styles, 146
Lecture, 144
Level of assistance, 65
    and when to use them, 66t
    decision-making guide, 67f–68
Librium, 83
Lighting, 30
    bathing room, 107–108
Live oak institute, 127
Looped drawsheet transfer, 102, 103f
Lotion, 90

Massage, 81
Mayday pain project, 85
McGill pain questionnaire, 76
McGill present pain intensity questionnaire, 76t–77
Mechanical lifts, 92, 117
Memory, 28
Meperidine, 83
Meprobamate, 83
Mesh seats, 118
Metamucil, 82
Miltown, 83
Mint bath, 81
Mirrors, 37–39
Modeling/gesturing, 68, 72, 74

Modesty, 43
Mood, 18, 26
    assessment, 22
Motor functioning, 28
Music, 37–38
    bathing room, 108

Noise, 25–27, 42
    of bathing room, 108
Non-narcotic analgesics, 82
Nonsteroidal anti-inflammatory drugs, 2, 82
Nonverbal signs of discomfort/pain, 77t
No-rinse shampoos, 120t
Norton, LaVrene, 127
Nurses
    changing role of, 129–130
Nursing assistant, 129

Occasional physical guidance, 68, 73, 74
Odors, 30
    bathing room
        elimination of, 108–109
Offer specific reinforcement, 72
Ointments, 82, 84
Older people, pain and related medications to avoid,
    83t, 84
Olfactory environment
    of bathing room, 108–109
One-step commands, 71–72
One-step verbal commands, 68
Oral tardive dyskinesia, 78
Organizational environment
    cultural change, 133–134
Organizational factors
    change process, 126
    decision-making
        direct care staff, 128–129
        resident, 128–129
Osteoporosis, 75

Paid care providers
    self-care, 164–165
Pain, 75
    assessment of nonverbal signs, 78
    description, 77–78
    unique expressions of, 78
Pain during bathing, minimizing interventions,
    80–84
    complementary treatments, 81
    nonmedication treatments, 80–84
    timing the medication, 82, 84
Pain medication trial step ladder, 79, 80t,
    81–82
Pain medications, 79–82

MONKLANDS HOSPITAL
LIBRARY
MONKSCOURT AVENUE
AIRDRIE ML60JS
☎ 01236712005